DISSEMINATING RESEARCH / CHANGING PRACTICE

RESEARCH METHODS FOR PRIMARY CARE

Series Board of Editors

The goal of RESEARCH METHODS FOR PRIMARY CARE is to address important topics meeting the needs of the growing number of primary care researchers. Purposely following a sequence from general principles to specific techniques, implementation strategies, and dissemination, the series volumes each examine a particular aspect of primary care research, emphasizing actually conducting research in the real world. The well-known contributors bring an international, multidisciplinary perspective to the volumes, enhancing their usefulness to primary care researchers.

Volumes in the series:

1. **Primary Care Research: Traditional and Innovative Approaches**
   Edited by Peter G. Norton, Moira Stewart, Fred Tudiver, Martin J. Bass, and Earl V. Dunn

2. **Tools for Primary Care Research**
   Edited by Moira Stewart, Fred Tudiver, Martin J. Bass, Earl V. Dunn, and Peter G. Norton

3. **Doing Qualitative Research: Multiple Strategies**
   Edited by Benjamin F. Crabtree and William L. Miller

4. **Assessing Interventions: Traditional and Innovative Methods**
   Edited by Fred Tudiver, Martin J. Bass, Earl V. Dunn, Peter G. Norton, and Moira Stewart

5. **Conducting Research in the Practice Setting**
   Edited by Martin J. Bass, Earl V. Dunn, Peter G. Norton, Moira Stewart, and Fred Tudiver

6. **Disseminating Research/Changing Practice**
   Edited by Earl V. Dunn, Peter G. Norton, Moira Stewart, Fred Tudiver, and Martin J. Bass

Disseminating Research / Changing Practice

EDITED BY

EARL V. DUNN
PETER G. NORTON
MOIRA STEWART
FRED TUDIVER
MARTIN J. BASS

Research Methods
for Primary Care
Volume 6

SAGE Publications
International Educational and Professional Publisher
Thousand Oaks   London   New Delhi

Copyright © 1994 by Sage Publications, Inc.

For information address:

SAGE Publications, Inc.
2455 Teller Road
Thousand Oaks, California 91320

SAGE Publications Ltd.
6 Bonhill Street
London EC2A 4PU
United Kingdom

SAGE Publications India Pvt. Ltd.
M-32 Market
Greater Kailash I
New Delhi 110 048 India

Printed in the United States of America

Library of Congress Cataloging-in-Publication Data

Main entry under title:

Disseminating research — changing practice / edited by Earl V. Dunn
. . . [et al.].
      p.   cm. — (Research methods for primary care; v. 6)
   Includes bibliographical references and index.
   ISBN 0-8039-5705-X. — ISBN 0-8039-5706-8 (pbk.)
   1. Primary care (Medicine)—Research. 2. Communication in
medicine. I. Dunn, Earl V. II. Series.
   R852.D55 1994
   362.1'072—dc20   94-10317

94 95 96 97 10 9 8 7 6 5 4 3 2 1

Sage Production Editor: Diane S. Foster

Contents

Foreword

KERR LACHLAN WHITE

More than 4 years ago this landmark series on *Research Methods for Primary Care* was conceived. The present volume completes the cycle by discussing at length the many ethical, collegial, scientific, political, and technical issues involved in disseminating the results of primary care research. Virtually all industrialized countries, as well as those in the developing world, now recognize that primary care provides the essential clinical underpinning for any balanced and affordable health care system. New national and institutional commitments will ensure adequate numbers of appropriately trained general physicians and strengthen substantially the relevant academic departments. The need has never been greater, therefore, to advise practitioners, the public, and politicians about new knowledge that impinges on the earliest manifestations of illness or that promotes good health.

Why has the public insisted on these changes in medicine's priorities, and why have politicians acted so vigorously? They have done so because individuals and populations demand prompt and effective responses to their real and perceived health problems. Health personnel—physicians, nurses, and other professionals—require useful, credible, and timely knowledge in order to respond appropriately. Explosions in telecommunications and information technologies are accelerating the real-time acquisition, storage, and transmission of this knowledge but, on balance, the clinical aspects of medical care—as distinguished from accounting and billing aspects—have been slow to benefit from opportunities these technological revolutions provide. Much of what follows in this volume is concerned with measures to accelerate application of these opportunities, especially as they apply to primary care practice.

Dissemination is after all only a fancy word that means "spread." All who carry out medical research of any kind have a solemn obligation to "spread the word." The tradition that requires investigators to report research findings to their peers in scientific journals is, for the most part, well observed. Frequently, however, investigators' accomplishments are modest when it comes to seeing that useful and usable knowledge stemming from their research is actually applied clinically to all patients who can benefit. Practices and policies that accurately inform the public and its politicians about research results are uneven. This is especially true for findings that can improve primary care practice. Compassionate, "evidence-based," affordable, and timely responses are what people—individually and collectively—want and need and what suitably prepared primary care and other practitioners strive to provide. The present volume includes discussions of this essential link in closing the loop from each patient's initial problems to their satisfactory resolution. Research results lying dormant in medical journals—esoteric or otherwise—or public pronouncements laced with jargon are unhelpful in achieving this objective. Without accurate and lucid exposition reflected in the media's reporting of new knowledge, the public fails to benefit from the research and scholarship it has supported, and the practicing professions' responses may too often be deficient.

The extensive set of observations and analyses to be found in the ensuing chapters should benefit both seasoned investigators and tyros. I want to dwell on one aspect of clinical investigation that is especially intriguing, however. Vivek Goel and C. David Naylor pose the problem bluntly in Chapter 16 when they write: "Much of the clinical research enterprise in industrialized nations addresses questions that appear at first glance to be almost wilfully irrelevant." I agree with this assessment and suggest that every medical school should conduct an extensive inventory of its clinical research to document clearly the patient care problem or question that each study purports to address. The inventory should include estimates of the approximate number of persons in the country or the world who might benefit from a useful outcome from the research, when they might expect to benefit, and at what cost. Such information is of keen interest to the public that does the suffering and pays the bills. The findings of each medical school's survey should be widely disseminated in the public media.

The same inventory should, of course, be conducted for primary care research. My suspicion is that too much of contemporary primary care research also deals with trivial, irrelevant, and ephemeral epiphenomena that may not merit dissemination—especially to the public. In my view, primary care research has yet to reach its full potential in exploring the submerged part of the iceberg of interacting forces and factors that culminate in health or disease. Few academic departments concerned with attracting and preparing general physicians have begun to investigate the origins and natural history of the diverse conditions, complaints, symptoms, and problems brought by individuals and populations to sources of primary care. Thanks to this volume and the five others in the series, primary care investigators everywhere have ready access to a wide range of quantitative and qualitative methods that extend far beyond the limited armamentarium used in most bench laboratories. But methods without the questions are of limited value.

Important problems, separated into researchable questions, that can be addressed in a feasible fashion are the hallmarks of sound clinical research. An "important" problem is one that affects large numbers of people, is associated with many days of disability and work or school loss, involves much pain and suffering, or requires the expenditure of large sums of money. A "researchable" question is one that has a reasonable prospect of being answered in the proposed study. Most large problems have to be divided into manageable units; like eating an elephant, it is best done one bite at a time. We should also avoid trivial approaches to global problems and global approaches to trivial problems. A "feasible" question is one that can be successfully pursued with the personnel, facilities, resources, and time available to the investigator. Curiosity, imagination, persistence, and courage are other criteria that characterize the first-rate investigator.

As this volume and its companions attest, the primary care establishment has a growing cadre of highly talented investigators equipped with a wide spectrum of, for the most part, established research methods suited to the equally broad array of problems and questions encountered in primary care practice. What is needed now is to stimulate students, faculty colleagues, and practitioners by applications that demonstrate how active clinical, practice-based, and population-based primary care research is at last following the examples set by those heroes of all primary care physicians and researchers—Sir James Mackenzie of Burnley and William Pickles of Wensleydale.

The high road for health care and medicine in the 21st century may well belong to primary care—but only when its research equals in quality and relevance the outstanding advances provided by the best biomedical and behavioral research conducted during the 20th century. Primary care will assume its rightful place when its practices are supported by exemplary research directed at people's earliest health and medical problems, and when its findings are disseminated rapidly and accurately. This volume and the entire series show us the way.

Acknowledgments

The editors would like to thank their colleagues at the Departments of Family Medicine at the Sunnybrook Health Science Centre and the University of Western Ontario for their patience and understanding while this endeavor was underway. The authors of the individual chapters were tolerant and helpful and did a remarkable job of adhering to our relatively stringent guidelines and deadlines. Anne Stilman did her usual excellent work in the editing of the manuscripts. Vanessa Orr spent considerable time and concentrated effort on the index. Most important, Jamie Jensen coordinated the schedule for the book, badgered the authors, typed and retyped manuscripts and kept the project on track. To all these individuals we are grateful.

The Physicians' Services Incorporated Foundation, Toronto, Ontario, and the National Health Research and Development Program (NHRDP) of the Federal Government of Canada provided financial assistance that made this project possible.

Introduction

EARL V. DUNN

Research findings are of little benefit to patients or to society if they do not reach the practitioner and if they are not implemented into practice. Thus dissemination of new knowledge and changing practitioner behavior are essential to the whole research process. Previous volumes in this series have followed the process of primary care research: formulating questions, techniques, and tools; qualitative methods; methods to assess interventions; and techniques that allow research in the community setting. This volume addresses the issues of ensuring that the new knowledge derived from research will be disseminated and will have an impact upon practice.

The stage is set in the initial chapter, which reviews the various theories of dissemination and change methods and advances an implementation model that gives us an understanding of the dissemination process and serves as a foundation for many of the remaining presentations in the volume. Following this chapter, the volume is divided into three parts that relate to dissemination, special topics, and changing behavior, respectively.

The first part addresses dissemination of primary care research. Its five chapters discuss different aspects of the dissemination process, including communications, ethics, and dissemination to other researchers, practitioners, and the public. The final chapter in this section presents a number of preliminary guidelines for primary care research dissemination, which were developed as part of the fifth Foundations of Primary Care Research conference, held in Toronto in February 1993.

The second section discusses methodological issues related to dissemination and to having an impact on practice. Two chapters address how to carry out dissemination research and how to assess impact, and the third reflects on the question of dissemination prior to peer review.

The final section examines, in detail, ways to change practitioner behavior. The first chapter here reviews the literature and highlights the evidence for the effectiveness of strategies for dissemination and behavior change. The six chapters that follow discuss various methods and strategies that have been used to impact on practitioner behavior. The topics addressed include clinical guidelines, evidence-based clinical practice, direct support for the practitioner, and affecting policy making. All are presented with specific implementation strategies and are illustrated with practical examples for primary care.

The volume concludes with an appendix that outlines tips on using the media to assist in dissemination of new knowledge. It addresses ways to optimally use the news release and methods for dealing with media representatives in different situations.

We hope that this volume, in conjunction with the others in the series, will assist primary care researchers in their endeavors. In particular, we expect that it will help all researchers to disseminate their findings. In spreading new knowledge, the researcher will accomplish the ultimate goal of clinical research—that is, to incorporate new findings into practice for the benefit of the patient and of society.

1 Teaching Old (and Not so Old) Docs New Tricks: Effective Ways to Implement Research Findings

JONATHAN LOMAS

Shortcomings and Persistence of Traditional Educational Approaches

It's a hectic afternoon in the family physician's office. The first three patient bookings are for a Mr. White, a Ms. Black, and a Mr. Grey. Dr. Decisive calls in 52-year-old Mr. White, who is seeing her for a follow-up visit to resolve complaints of irritability and mood swings. The test results indicate hyperthyroidism; the extremely high probability of a successful outcome from radioactive iodine treatment is discussed, and Mr. White is referred for the procedure.

Ms. Black is next. She is 22 weeks pregnant and wishes to have another ultrasound—she already had one at 17 weeks—to allay her concerns that "something is wrong with the baby." The inability of ultrasound to detect or demonstrate some new abnormality at 22 weeks is pointed out and, after an uneventful examination and some reassuring discussion, she leaves with no further intervention planned.

Finally, Mr. Grey enters the office, in a somewhat agitated state, with his 5-year-old boy who is complaining of earache for the third

AUTHOR'S NOTE: The author receives support from the Ontario Ministry of Health as a Career Scientist. Thank you to the Polinomics Research Group at McMaster University and to Brian Hutchison for comments on an earlier version of this chapter.

1

time this winter. Upon examination it is clear that the ear is red. Dr. Decisive is concerned about the recurring nature of these episodes and about their potential long-term harm. The child is already on prophylactic antibiotics, but what about considering tubes? Dr. Decisive discusses the pros and cons with Mr. Grey, points out that her colleagues are divided on the value of tubes for resolving persistent otitis media and, feeling unsatisfied, writes a prescription for a course of another antibiotic and agrees to "wait and see what happens."

The focus of those investigating the implementation of research findings has been very much on the Mr. Whites and Ms. Blacks of this world. Yet the average family physician's practice is full of Mr. Greys—symptom presentations where the physician is uncertain what, if any, intervention to undertake. In some of our own work on cesarean section, a panel doing independent ratings could not agree on the advisability of surgical intervention for 62% of the possible clinical presentations. Even after convening and discussing it as a group, they still failed to reach agreement on 53% of presentations (Lomas et al., 1988). Similarly, in a recent study of red blood cell transfusion practices, Soumerai et al. (1993) found that up to one third of the cases fell into a category where there was "a high degree of disagreement within the medical community about the indications for transfusion in these patients" (p. 962).

In other words, much of the time physicians engage in "informed guesswork" when it comes to prescribing or not prescribing particular interventions. Perhaps this is what we mean when we talk of the "art of medicine." What, then, is used by the physician to inform the guesses? If so much of medical decision making is not considered black and white, but is like the informed guess for Mr. Grey and his 5-year-old, something more than research findings is clearly playing an important role in informing patient care decisions. Much of the research on physician behavior has, however, ignored this discretionary area where these other influential factors are most likely to be observable. It has focused instead on studying the behavior of physicians when the clinical situation is perceived to be black (clear absence of indications for intervention) or white (unambiguous presence of indications for intervention).

These black and white areas are, by definition, where a research study is so clear and unambiguous that it compels attention and is therefore very likely to be highly influential on practice. For example, when the randomized controlled trial (RCT) results showing the ineffectiveness of extracranial/intracranial arterial bypass surgery for stroke prevention were released, there was an immediate and marked reduction in the use of this procedure. This is not to say that *all* EC/IC bypass surgery ceased; only that the research finding had a major impact. But what does the average GP do when asked by a 50-year-old woman whether she should embark on regular mammography for early detection of breast cancer? The latest Canadian study (Miller, Baines, To, & Wall, 1992) might well deter such a recommendation, but how should this be weighed against the previous four studies in the area that would encourage it (Andersson et al., 1988; Roberts et al., 1990; Shapiro, Venet, Strax, Venet, & Roeser, 1982; Tabar et al., 1985)?

By focusing so much on what happens in the compelling black and white areas, investigators have tended to overemphasize the role of relatively passive education in influencing physician decision making. Because the focus has been on the compelling research findings, the belief persists that publication in a journal, supplemented by a few continuing medical education sessions, is usually enough to flow the results into practice. It is clear, however, that even an apparently black or white educational message can be overpowered by such influences as inertia, peer pressure, economic advantage, malpractice concern, or pharmaceutical marketing. But this is hardly surprising if these influences are justifiably relied upon to fill the void left by absent, uncertain, or contradictory research findings that define all the grey areas of medical practice.

Thus the first conclusion might be that if you look under the lamppost you will find that which is obvious (education may effectively implement compelling research findings) but miss the key (most of the time education is not enough). Many of the implications from research, although black and white to the researcher, are not immediately compelling to the practitioner, whose clinical decision making therefore continues as if he or she were in the discretionary grey area. Indeed, the popularity and importance of RCTs is largely attributable to the fact that most of the effects of new interventions are so subtle that only carefully controlled and unbiased investigations can pick out the small effects from the natural and random fluctuations in outcome. (Most recently the use of meta-analyses has enabled such subtle effects to be revealed at an earlier date; see Lau et al., 1992.) There are few "aha's" such as penicillin left to be discovered and reported upon.

The work of Greer and other sociologists interviewing community physicians reveals one of the major consequences of this state of affairs (Clark, Potter, & McKinlay, 1991; Greer, 1988). Research findings hold no special value to the local physician; they are just another one of the many inputs that may or may not determine the final practice decision. These studies highlight the importance of the local community's norms, built up over long periods of sustained day-to-day contact, in determining practice decisions. Research findings may contribute, but the views of an influential local colleague or discussion in the surgical locker-room are likely to carry at least as much if not more weight. It is not surprising, therefore, to find that traditional continuing medical education (Davis, Thomson, Oxman, & Haynes, 1992; Haynes, Davis, McKibbon, & Tugwell, 1984), the dissemination of printed materials (Avorn & Soumerai, 1983; Evans, Haynes, & Birkett, 1986), and even the release of authoritative practice guidelines (Kosecoff et al., 1987; Lomas et al., 1989) have little or no impact on practice behaviors.

Despite these findings, the organized structures of the medical profession continue to rely largely upon traditional passive education as the main mechanism for the attempted transfer of research into practice. In a recent survey of 11 medical profession organizations in Canada concerned with obstetrical care, 2 had no planned activities to bring new research to the attention of obstetrical practitioners, and the remaining 9 had no activities in place or planned beyond newsletters, CME conferences, or task force investigations and reports. Even among a further 27 administrator, consumer, or government organizations involved with obstetrical care, only one was actually using or planned to use more aggressive implementation efforts such as chart audits or advertising and marketing campaigns (Lomas, 1993). This is despite the recent availability of a carefully synthesized body of obstetrical research within the covers of *Effective Care in Pregnancy and Childbirth* (Chalmers, Enkin, & Keirse, 1989). Most saw the publication and availability of this innovative text as all that was necessary for its implications to become incorporated into practice.

Systematic investigations of the routes and sources of influence on professional decision making are available. These investigations, often grounded in the approaches and methods of disciplines outside medicine, could inform the professional organizations of medicine should they wish to develop programs that help Dr. Decisive fully exploit existing research findings, at least when dealing with the Mr. Whites and Ms. Blacks of her practice. Successfully developing such programs would restrict the grey area, where medical discretion is exercised and tolerated, to only those clinical decisions for which research was truly unavailable, contradictory, or inapplicable. The next section reviews four alternatives to passive education and isolates principles for the design of such physician behavior change initiatives.

Approaches to Understanding
Physician Behavior Change

Lessons about how to flow research findings into practice can be extracted from the social influences literature, studies of the diffusion of innovations, adult learning theory, and marketing approaches.

SOCIAL INFLUENCES MODEL

The social influences model has its roots in psychology and sociology and the concept of local norms. "The behavioral models of decision-making underlying the social influence perspective holds that peers' judgement and beliefs play a major role in an individual's evaluation of new information" (Mittman, Tonesk, & Jacobson, 1992, p. 414). In contrast to traditional passive education views of physician behavior change, social influence approaches point to habit, socially accepted norms of appropriateness, and peer acceptance as the motivators for change, rather than such rational motives as cost-benefit analyses and imputed impacts on patient outcomes. Modeling behavior as a member of a social group takes precedence over acquiring and applying information as an isolated individual.

DIFFUSION OF INNOVATIONS LITERATURE

The second area, studies on the diffusion of innovations, has largely been the domain of sociologists such as Coleman and colleagues (Coleman, Katz, & Menzel, 1966; Greer, 1988; Rogers, 1983; Stocking, 1985). By observing how medical innovations actually find their way into local practice, these investigators have highlighted three important considerations.

First, the closed nature of most medical communities and the importance of local product champions and opinion leaders is noted: "The central theme of medical diffusion studies is that physicians act as communities rather than aggregates of unrelated individuals and that medical behavior is literally contagious" (Dixon, 1990, p. 208).

Second, they focus on the dynamic nature of diffusion wherein modification and adaptation to the local circumstances occur as part of a staged process of adoption: "If the innovation is defined too explicitly with too many restrictions on its modification, then its diffusion may be hindered" (Stocking, 1985, p. 75).

Third, and in contrast to the social influences model, diffusion theory isolates important characteristics of an innovation (rather than the practitioner's environment) that influence the diffusion process: its "relative advantage" (for the adoptee and for patient care), its "compatibility" (with personal and local norms), its "complexity," its "trialability" (extent to which it can be tried temporarily and discarded if found wanting), and its "observability" (how easily one can see whether the expected results are being achieved) have been identified (Rogers, 1983). In recent empirical work we have confirmed the importance of at least the complexity and trialability (but not observability) of 143 clinical recommendations extracted from practice guidelines in predicting compliance or adoption by physicians (Grilli & Lomas, 1994).

ADULT LEARNING THEORY

Adult learning theory also focuses on the characteristics of the expected behavior change (or innovation) as well as of the practitioner's environment. Based on interviews with 356 physicians, Fox, Mazmanian, and Putnam (1989) highlight the importance of personal motivation rather than coercion in achieving sustained behavior change. They note that "learning sometimes . . . was used to help prepare to change, and to verify that the change was positive and valuable" (p. 174). Education and the consequent learning are not, therefore, useless; they contribute to predisposing practitioners to consider change and reinforce that change once it has occurred: however, they rarely enable the actual change (Green & Eriksen, 1988).

MARKETING APPROACHES

Finally, physician behavior change is now being addressed by marketing approaches, following the development of social marketing techniques to sell health promotion to the general public (Kotler & Roberto, 1989). Many of the principles for this approach are derived from advertising and the literature on persuasive communication: "It distinguishes five attributes of communication that are consistently important: the 'source' or originator of the communication; . . . the 'channel' or medium of presentation; the 'message' content itself; the characteristics of the 'audience' receiving the communication; and finally, the 'setting' in which the communication is received" (Winkler, Lohr, & Brook, 1985, pp. 314-315). This literature also makes a distinction between communications that merely increase awareness and those that may actually bring about changes in behavior. The latter consist of a more restricted set of influences that focus on influentials as the source, personalized interactions as the channel, local anecdote or experience as the message, opinion leaders as the audience, and informal environments as the setting. It is noteworthy that few, if any, of these considerations are to be found in the traditional educational communication of research findings, although most are found in the promotional and marketing efforts of pharmaceutical companies (Avorn, Chen, & Hartley, 1982).

Each of these four approaches makes both unique and common contributions to our understanding of how research findings might influence physician behavior. A focus on social influences underlines the need to view physicians as members of small, locally based, and closed medical communities in which research findings must find resonance with existing norms and values. Studies on the diffusion of innovations also emphasize the importance of the local medical community and its influentials, but in addition draw attention to the need to design modifiable messages from the research that can be adapted to fit the local environment. Adult learning theory highlights the need for the physician to be predisposed to accept change before efforts are made to implement research findings; that is, behavior change is a dynamic process, not an overnight event or a coercive act. Finally, the marketing literature once again stresses the value of using local agents-for-change as the source of the research message, as well as ensuring that the message itself is designed to appeal to the concerns of the target physician.

The physician is, therefore, not a tabula rasa waiting to be informed. He or she has existing experience, beliefs, practice policies, and habits, and these are reinforced by the numerous routes of influence in the local environment. Common to all four of the approaches reviewed above is the message that physicians are subject to powerful and potentially determining influences in their local environments. In broad terms, these influences are mapped in the "Coordinated Implementation Model" of Figure 1.1 as educational, administrative, personal, patient based, community based, and economic. The figure highlights the extent to which the practitioner is embedded in a powerful local network of influences. Even with research information that has been synthesized and disseminated by a credible body, its impact is likely to go no further than the awareness, attitude, and knowledge of the physician if the historical focus on just the educational route of influence (the "shadow boxes" in Figure 1.1) is maintained. Finding ways to ensure that the research information flows as freely through the other routes of influence as it does through the educational route will significantly enhance the probability of successful implementation through changes in the behavior of the physician.

In summary, research findings are most likely to find their way into practice when most or all of the following conditions hold:

The Message and Its Source

- The research is synthesized by a credible and influential body and packaged in a "user friendly" format with a message that justifies the need for change by comparison with existing approaches, norms and concerns: that is, it is a persuasive communication.

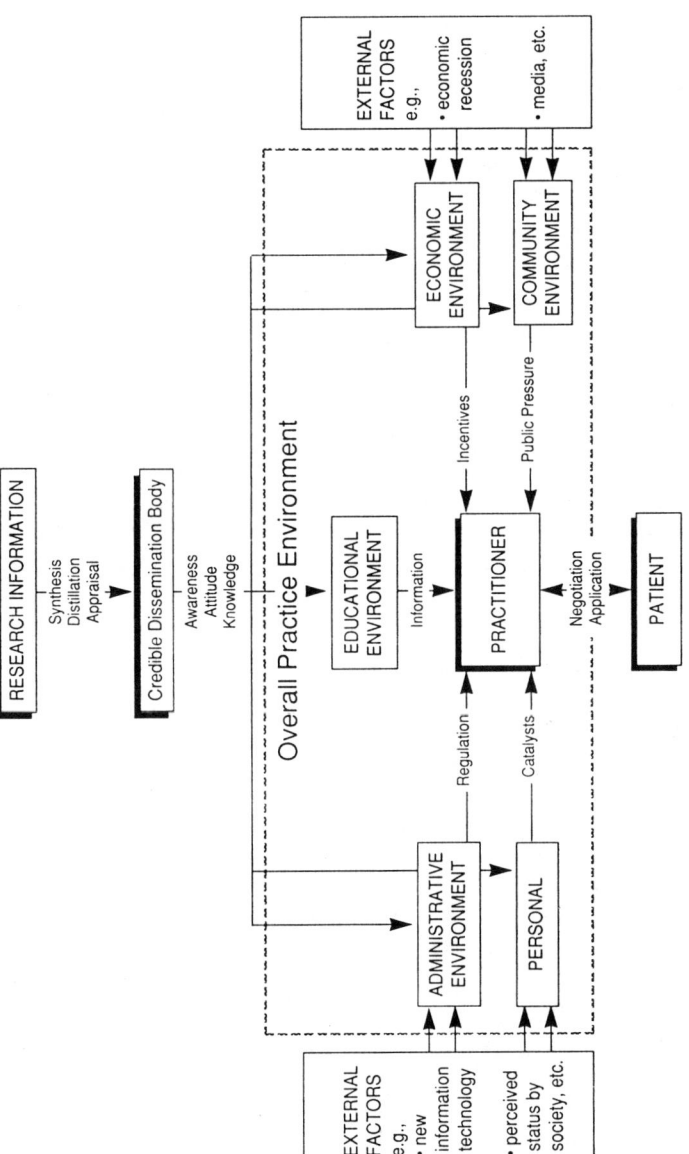

Figure 1.1. The Coordinated Implementation Model

SOURCE: Milbank Quarterly, 1993. 71(3), p. 445. Reprinted with permission.

- The implied change is implementable within flexible parameters and implementation is within the power of the target physician without the need for extensive collaboration and cooperation with others.

The Communication Channels

- The existence and importance of the research findings are communicated to the physician from a variety of sources that are both within and outside the local community.
- There are respected and influential local exemplars considering or actually adopting the findings for their own practices.

The Implementation Setting

- There is an opportunity to explore the implications of the research findings in a personal encounter with either an influential local colleague or a respected outside authority.
- Adoption of the findings will not come into conflict with the economic or administrative incentives of the physician's working environment, nor with the expectations of his or her patients or the communities from which they come.

Translating Principles Into Programs

Empirical validation of the largely theoretical propositions of the previous section can be found in a review of the relatively small number of positively evaluated interventions to implement research findings. With the burgeoning popularity of practice guidelines has come a parallel growth in the evaluation of methods for bringing about changes in physician behavior based upon the guidelines. I will not review all these evaluations here as a number of others have already undertaken such reviews (e.g., Agency for Health Care Policy and Research, 1992; Davis et al., 1992; Eisenberg, 1986; Grol, 1992; Lomas & Haynes, 1988; Mittman et al., 1992; Schroeder, 1987; Stafford, 1990; Stocking, 1992). Rather, I will select intervention programs that appear to hold the most promise for implementing research findings, and tie their contents back to the principles outlined above.

This type of research is, however, still at an early enough stage of development to believe that the programs listed below by no means exhaust the possibilities for successful research implementation strategies. Many other creative combinations and applications of the principles are likely possible. Finally, and recalling the black, white, and grey world of medical decision making highlighted in the introduction, such sophisticated programs are of most use in those areas of practice where, despite the availability of research that indicates a black or white choice, clinical discretion still reigns as if the decision area were grey. The more traditional forms of education and dissemination may often suffice for those few black or white decisions where the research is so compelling that the competing social, economic, and administrative influences can be overpowered by information transmission alone.

OPINION LEADERS AND EDUCATIONAL INFLUENTIALS

Recruiting locally designated opinion leaders or educational influentials to organize and encourage implementation of a particular research finding in their community has proven effective in a number of evaluations (e.g., Lomas et al., 1991; Stross & Bole, 1980). Most often these recruits are provided with a brief orientation to the research findings, possibly equipped with printed educational materials, and left to undertake whatever activities they deem necessary to achieve implementation in their community. This strategy is explicitly focused on the importance of the local community's norms, the orientation of practitioners to locally credible individuals, and the need to translate the research findings into a locally applicable message.

ACADEMICALLY BASED DETAILING

Face-to-face personal and interactive visits with an outside expert, who is equipped with printed materials and information on the likely general concerns of the target physician, and who is able to provide concrete strategies to implement the research findings have proved effective in bringing about behavior change (e.g., Avorn & Soumerai, 1983; Ray, Blazer, Schaffner, Federspiel, & Fink, 1986). The components of these "educational outreach" programs (Soumerai & Avorn, 1990) address both the need for messages to be congruent with physicians' existing beliefs and concerns, and the power of a personal encounter with a credible source who provides easily understood materials and practical advice.

REMINDER SYSTEMS

With the widespread availability of computer technology, especially in the hospital environment, incorporating reminders into the documentation and prescribing systems of a physician's environment has become both feasible and, apparently, effective as an implementation strategy (e.g., Haynes & Walker, 1987; Murrey, Gottlieb, & Schoenbaum, 1992). It is often the case that the affected physicians contribute to the design of both the reminder's contents and to its operation within the system of care (Gottlieb, Margolis, & Schoenbaum, 1990; Spiegel, Shapiro, Berman, & Greenfield, 1989). To a large degree this strategy enables the message to be personalized and tailored to the local community, as well as incorporated into the incentives of the physician's administrative environment.

CONTINUOUS QUALITY IMPROVEMENT

There has been an almost religious conversion of many health-care facilities to the industrial-quality management process of continuous quality improvement (CQI). CQI involves the application of principles that recognize individuals as components of a system, and views these systems, rather than the individuals, as the unit of analysis in identifying barriers and developing solutions to the implementation of research findings (Kritchevsky & Simmons, 1991). Evaluations of this approach are encouraging about its ability to flow research findings into organized institutional settings such as hospitals and health maintenance organizations (e.g., Burns et al., 1992). Caution is warranted, however, until less passionate (and potentially more objective) investigations of its effectiveness are undertaken once the gloss of "latest panacea" has worn off—health services researchers can succumb as easily as physicians to over-diffusion via the lure of the latest technology! Nevertheless, CQI does incorporate many of the principles of a successful behavior-change initiative, especially with its focus on administrative as well as educational incentives and the recognition of the physician as a fallible member of a local system.

MEDIA MARKETING

There are several examples of effective use of the popular media, supplemented by professional messages, to communicate and implement research findings. One study used local media to reduce the use of hysterectomy (Domenighetti et al., 1988); another used the national media to communicate the association between Reye's syndrome and aspirin in children (Soumerai, Ross-Degnan, & Kahn, 1992). Directly targeting the public, especially with messages that are easily understood, multiplies the routes of communication, encourages physician-patient discussions, and likely generates debate between colleagues in a community.

OTHER METHODS

There are two perhaps surprising omissions from this listing of potential programs—economic incentives and audit with feedback. Although economic incentives can undoubtedly generate changes in physician behavior, they have been omitted as a program here because "behaviour can be changed irrespective of evidence about clinical benefit. Because the underlying intention is that clinicians should base their practice on scientific evidence, using financial incentives can have the negative byproduct of discouraging practitioners to think about their practice" (Stocking, 1992, p. 59).

With regard to audit with feedback, there are some examples of putatively successful interventions, but these are balanced by an almost equivalent number of failures (Davis et al., 1992). Reviewing this literature, Eisenberg (1986) states that these programs "are most likely to be successful if the data are individualized, if doctors are compared with their peers, and if the information is delivered personally by a physician in a position of clinical leadership" (p. 117). Scrutiny of the characteristics of the successes and failures leads one to the working hypothesis that it is not audit and feedback per se that are effective, but rather that success is dependent upon incorporating a local opinion leader (e.g., Myers & Gleicher, 1988), or a reminder system (e.g., Mugford, Banford, & O'Hanlan, 1991) as the feedback element.

Finally, none of these programs is likely to be successful if operated in a vacuum with no prior "predisposing" activities to make physicians aware of the information and prepare them to consider changes in practice. It is here that the increasing availability of practice guidelines acts as a complement to the potentially enabling strategies listed in this section. Similarly, other influences from outside the local community, such as the expectations of and communications by professional licensing and competence assessment bodies, or the messages from litigation outcomes, will influence the willingness of physicians in a local community to undertake the effort of incorporating potentially disruptive implications of research findings into their practices. Ultimately, however, the incorporation of a particular research finding into a particular physician's practice is dependent upon how much one is able to generate resonance for the findings in that physician's closed and local medical community: "In all communities the 'results' which the majority are watching are not in the distant and confusing findings of the literature but those in their local communities" (Greer, 1988, p. 12).

Even when programs are in place that successfully generate such resonance in the local community for useful and valid research findings, they will only have maximized the size of the black and white areas of the clinical decision. There will still remain a substantial proportion of Mr. Greys in the physician's practice. Help for Dr. Decisive with these cases is further away. The research community has tended to generate information for her under the assumption that a definitive "black and white" answer can eventually be found. Dr. Decisive may not agree, confronted as she is with the grey of what researchers call "confounding" variables—variations in local skill and expertise, uneven availability of facilities and, perhaps most important, idiosyncratic patient preferences for particular risk and benefit trade-offs. For the circumstances where these confounders prevail, current research, focusing as it does on finding the one correct intervention, is unlikely to be helpful.

What would help with these grey decisions is research that portrays the risks and benefits of all the options in an understandable form for both the physician and the patient. The decision for the physician is not which intervention to use, but what options to present to the patient and with what information to help him or her make a choice. It is not at all clear that researchers appreciate the importance of this kind of information to the practitioner. The use of research findings to improve decision making, or choices, in the grey area may depend more on a change in researchers' behavior than it does on changes in practitioners' behavior. The more the research is relevant to and helpful for the daily decision making of the community practitioner, the more likely it is to find its way into community practice.

References

Agency for Health Care Policy and Research. (1992). *Annotated bibliography, effective dissemination to health care practitioners and policy makers* (AHCPR Pub. No. 92-0030). Washington, DC: Author.

Andersson, I., Aspegren, K., Janzon, L., Landberg, T., Lindholm, K., Linell, F., Ljungberg, O., Ranstam, J., & Sigfesson, B. (1988). Mammographic screening and mortality from breast cancer: The Malmo mammographic screening trial. *British Medical Journal, 297,* 943-948.

Avorn, J., Chen, N., & Hartley, R. (1982). Scientific vs. commercial sources of influence on the prescribing behavior of physicians. *American Journal of Medicine, 73,* 4-8.

Avorn, J., & Soumerai, S. B. (1983). Improving drug-therapy decisions through educational outreach. *New England Journal of Medicine, 308,* 1457-1463.

Burns, L., Denton, M., Goldfein, S., Warrick, L., Morenz, B., & Sales, B. (1992, December). The use of continuous quality improvement methods in the development and dissemination of medical practice guidelines. *Quality Review Bulletin,* pp. 434-439.

Chalmers, I., Enkin, M., & Keirse, M. (1989). *Effective care in pregnancy and childbirth.* Oxford: Oxford University Press.

Clark, J. A., Potter, D. A., & McKinlay, J. B. (1991). Bringing social structure back into clinical decision making. *Social Science and Medicine, 32,* 853-866.

Coleman, J. S., Katz, E., & Menzel, H. (1966). *Medical innovation: A diffusion study.* Indianapolis, IN: Bobbs-Merrill.

Davis, D. A., Thomson, M. A., Oxman, A. D., & Haynes R. B. (1992). Evidence for the effectiveness of CME: A review of 50 randomized controlled trials. *Journal of the American Medical Association, 268*(9), 1111-1117.

Dixon, A. (1990). The evolution of clinical policies. *Medical Care, 28,* 201-220.

Domenighetti, G., Luraschi, P., Gutzwiller, F., Pedrinis, E., Casabianca, A., Spinelli, A., & Repetto, F. (1988, December 24/31). Effect of information campaign by the mass media on hysterectomy rates. *Lancet,* pp. 1470-1473.

Eisenberg, J. M. (1986). *Doctors' decisions and the costs of medical care*. Ann Arbor, MI: Health Administration Press.

Evans, C., Haynes, R., & Birkett, N. (1986). Does a mailed continuing education program improve physician performance? *Journal of the American Medical Association, 225*, 501-504.

Fox, R. D., Mazmanian, P. E., & Putnam, R. W. (1989). *Changing and learning in the lives of physicians*. New York: Praeger.

Gottlieb, L., Margolis, C., & Schoenbaum, S. (1990). Clinical practice guidelines at an HMO: Development and implementation in a quality improvement model. *Quality Review Bulletin, 16*, 80-86.

Green, L., & Eriksen, M. (1988). Behavioral determinants of preventive practices by physicians. *American Journal of Preventive Medicine, 4*(suppl.), 101-107.

Greer, A. L. (1988). The state of the art versus the state of the science: The diffusion of new medical technologies into practice. *International Journal of Technology Assessment in Health Care, 4*, 5-26.

Grilli, R., & Lomas, J. G. (1994). Evaluating the message: The relationship between compliance rate and the subject of a practice guideline. *Medical Care, 32*(3), 202-213.

Grol, R. (1992). Implementing guidelines in general practice care. *Quality in Health Care, 1*, 184-191.

Haynes, R. B., & Walker, C. (1987). Computer-aided quality assurance: A critical appraisal. *Archives of Internal Medicine, 147*, 1297-1301.

Haynes, R. B., Davis, D. A., McKibbon, A., & Tugwell, P. (1984). A critical appraisal of the efficacy of continuing medical education. *Journal of the American Medical Association, 251*(1), 61-64.

Kosecoff, J., Kanouse, D., Rogers, W., McCloskey, L., Winslow, C., & Brook, R. (1987). Effects of the National Institutes of Health Consensus Development Program on physician practice. *Journal of the American Medical Association, 258*, 2708-2713.

Kotler, P., & Roberto, E. (1989). *Social marketing: Strategies for changing public behavior*. New York: Free Press.

Kritchevsky, S. B., & Simmons, B. P. (1991). Continuous quality improvement: Concepts and applications for physician care. *Journal of the American Medical Association, 266*(13), 1817-1823.

Lau, J., Antman, E., Jimenez-Silva, J., Kupelnick, B., Mosteller, F., & Chalmers, T. (1992, July 23). Cumulative meta-analysis of therapeutic trials for myocardial infarction. *New England Journal of Medicine, 327*(4), 248-254.

Lomas, J. (1993). Retailing research: Increasing the role of evidence in clinical services for child birth. *The Milbank Quarterly, 71*, 439-475.

Lomas, J., Anderson, G. M., Enkin, M., Vayda, E., Roberts, R., & MacKinnon, B. (1988). The role of evidence in the consensus process: Results from a Canadian consensus exercise. *Journal of the American Medical Association, 259*(20), 3001-3005.

Lomas, J., Anderson, G. M., Dominick-Pierre, K., Vayda, E., Enkin, M. W., & Hannah, W. J. (1989). Do practice guidelines guide practice? The effect of a consensus statement on the practice of physicians. *New England Journal of Medicine, 321*(19), 1306-1311.

Lomas, J., Enkin, M., Anderson, G. M., Hannah, W. J., Vayda, E., & Singer, J. (1991). Opinion leaders vs. audit and feedback to implement practice guidelines. Delivery after previous cesarean section. *Journal of the American Medical Association, 265*(17), 2202-2207.

Lomas, J., & Haynes, R. (1988). A taxonomy and critical review of tested strategies for the application of clinical practice recommendations: From "official" to "individual" clinical policy. In R. N. Battista & R. S. Lawrence (Eds.), Implementing preventive services. *American Journal of Preventive Medicine, 4* (suppl.), 77-95.

Miller, A., Baines, C., To, T., & Wall, C. (1992). Canadian National Breast Screening Study: 2. Breast cancer detection and death rates among women aged 50 to 59 years. *Canadian Medical Association Journal, 147*(10), 1477-1488.

Mittman, B., Tonesk, X., & Jacobson, P. (1992, December). Implementing clinical practice guidelines: Social influence strategies and practitioner behavior change. *Quality Review Bulletin*, pp. 413-422.

Mugford, M., Banfield, P., & O'Hanlon, M. (1991). Effects of feedback of information on clinical practice: A review. *British Medical Journal, 303*, 398-402.

Murrey, K., Gottlieb, L., & Schoenbaum, S. (1992). Implementing clinical guidelines: A quality management approach to reminder systems. *Quality Review Bulletin, 18*, 423-433.

Myers, S., & Gleicher, N. (1988). A successful program to lower cesarean section rates. *New England Journal of Medicine, 319*(23), 151-156.

Ray, W., Blazer, D., Schaffner, W., Federspiel, C., & Fink, R. (1986). Reducing long-term diazepam prescribing in office practice: A controlled trial of education visits. *Journal of the American Medical Association, 256*, 2536-2539.

Roberts, M., Alexander, F., Anderson, T., Chetty, U., Donnan, P., Forrest, P., Hepburn, W., Huggins, A., Kirkpatrick, A., Lamb, J., Muir, B., & Prescott, R. (1990). Edinburgh trial of screening for breast cancer: Mortality at seven years. *Lancet, 335*, 241-246.

Rogers, E. M. (1983). *Diffusion of innovations* (3rd ed.). New York: Free Press.

Schroeder, S. (1987). Strategies for reducing medical costs by changing physicians' behaviour: Efficacy and impact on quality of care. *International Journal of Technology Assessment in Health Care, 3*, 39-50.

Shapiro, S., Venet, W., Strax, P., Venet, L., & Roeser, R. (1982). Ten- to fourteen-year effect of screening on breast cancer mortality. *Journal of the National Cancer Institute, 69*, 349-355.

Soumerai, S. B., & Avorn, J. (1990). Principles of educational outreach ("academic detailing") to improve clinical decision making. *Journal of the American Medical Association, 263*(4), 549-556.

Soumerai, S. B., Ross-Degnan, D., & Kahn, J. (1992). Effects of professional and media warnings about the association between aspirin use in children and Reye's syndrome. *The Milbank Quarterly, 70*, 155-182.

Soumerai, S. B., Salem-Schatz, S., Avorn, J., Casteris, C., Ross-Degnan, D., & Popovsky, M. (1993). A controlled trial of educational outreach to improve blood transfusion practice. *Journal of the American Medical Association, 270*(8), 961-966.

Spiegel, J. S., Shapiro, M. F., Berman, B., & Greenfield, S. (1989). Changing physician test ordering in a university hospital: An intervention of physician participation, explicit criteria, and feedback. *Archives of Internal Medicine, 149*(3), 549-553.

Stafford, R. (1990). Alternative strategies for controlling rising cesarean section rates. *Journal of the American Medical Association, 263*, 683-687.

Stocking, B. (1985). *Initiative and inertia. Case studies in the NHS.* London: The Nuffield Provincial Hospitals Trust.

Stocking, B. (1992). Promoting change in clinical care. *Quality in Health Care, 1*, 56-60.

Stross, J. K., & Bole, G. G. (1980). Evaluation of a continuing education program in rheumatoid arthritis. *Arthritis and Rheumatism, 23*, 846-849.

Tabar, L., Gad, A., Holmberg, L., Ljungquist, U., Fagerberg, C., Baldetorp, L., Grontoft, O., Lundstrom, B., Mansson, J., Eklund, G., Day, N., & Pettersson, F. (1985). Reduction in mortality from breast cancer after mass screening with mammography. Randomised trial from the Breast Cancer Screening Working Group of the Swedish National Board of Health and Welfare. *Lancet, 1*, 829-832.

Winkler, J., Lohr, K., & Brook, R. (1985). Persuasive communication and medical technology assessment. *Archives of Internal Medicine, 145*, 314-317.

PART I

General Aspects of Dissemination

2 From Science to Practice: The Evolving Art of Communication

RENALDO N. BATTISTA
EMILY A. C. RUIZ
AZANA N. ENDICOTT

In Hippocrates' time, the knowledge and the practice of healing were indistinguishable. In the 1990s, however, science and practice are two different worlds, due to the explosion of technological advancements made in the past 100 years. Health *science* can be defined as the body of knowledge that results from a spectrum of health-related research activities, including basic research, epidemiological and clinical epidemiological research, and health services research (Battista et al., 1989). Health *practice* is defined broadly to include a variety of health-oriented actions initiated by practitioners, policy makers, and the public.

The distance between science and practice has increased markedly. To produce a successful transfer of knowledge into practice, a variety of dissemination strategies supported by organizational incentives need to be initiated, involving researchers, practitioners, policy makers, the media, and the public. The key to a successful interaction among all these players is communication, defined by MacDonald (1986, p. 395) as "a process of exchanging information through the use of commonly understood symbols."

In this chapter we will attempt to delineate some of these complex communication networks and provide examples that illustrate the dynamics of communication in bringing knowledge into effective practice.

Communication Among Researchers

Communication is central to the academic community, because both the promotion of knowledge (the cognitive concern) and the establishment of reputations (the social concern) depend on it (Becher, 1989).

Within a single discipline, communication among scientists is facilitated by a common understanding of terminology and, more importantly, because they share the same "constellation of beliefs, values, [and] techniques," defined by Kuhn (1970, p. 175) as a *paradigm*. Between disciplines, however, communication can be thwarted by differences of paradigm.

Interdisciplinarity refers to the synthesis of two or more disciplines, establishing a new meta-level of discourse, as opposed to *multidisciplinarity*, the juxtaposition of disciplines in an additive but not integrative fashion (Klein, 1990, pp. 55-73). A drive toward interdisciplinary interaction has accelerated in recent years, because given the complexity of scientific fields and of society, problems cannot be addressed by a single discipline or by individual experts (Haltery, 1986). Furthermore, as certain disciplines reach their limits in answering specific research questions through the application of their own theories and techniques, borrowing those developed in a different discipline may be very useful (Luszki, 1958).

The need to synthesize the rapidly increasing knowledge in the health field has triggered the development of a variety of approaches and techniques that combine information from multiple sources to establish "the state of science" on specific health care interventions, and to formulate recommendations for practicing clinicians and policy makers.

One such approach is the use of consensus conferences, in which a panel of members from different disciplines attempts first to decode scientific information presented by expert speakers and then to produce a synthesis document that captures the essence of their debate (McGlynn, Kosecoff, & Brook, 1990).

Other, more explicit approaches use a rating scheme to evaluate the efficacy and effectiveness of interventions, by assessing the strength of the scientific evidence documented in individual studies. A good example of this approach is the one developed by the Canadian Task Force on the Periodic Health Examination (1979), and later adopted by the U.S. Preventive Services Task Force (1989). The Canadian Task Force was innovative in clearly distinguishing two steps in the consensus process. The first phase grades the evidence, giving more weight to pieces of evidence derived from stronger research designs; this information is then sifted by a panel of experts who integrate other dimensions such as ethical considerations, cost issues, accessibility, acceptability, and safety, in order to formulate a specific recommendation (Woolf et al., 1990).

Whether the synthesis exercise proceeds through implicit rules or through a more structured approach, such as the one promoted by the Canadian Task Force on the Periodic Health Examination, the process brings scientists from a variety of backgrounds together to exchange points of view and to enter into debate in order to establish the state of health science.

An illustration of how researchers' disciplinary backgrounds may affect their approach to achieving the same goal is shown in Figure 2.1, which deals with understanding the causal pathway leading to recommendations on the early detection of high serum cholesterol levels (Battista & Fletcher, 1988). Basic scientists would focus more on experimental data demonstrating the capacity for early detection interventions to correctly identify high serum cholesterol levels (link 1) and for interventions to successfully decrease these levels (link 2), whereas epidemiologists would demand proof that cholesterol screening will ultimately decrease mortality from coronary heart disease (link 5) if not total mortality.

Communication Between Researchers and Practitioners

The ultimate objective of communicating scientific information to clinical practitioners is to help them improve the quality of health care delivered to the population. This communication is done through different channels.

One important source of information for practitioners is print communication. Scientific journals often have the additional objective of being a forum for exchanging information among researchers; however, this literature can be so complex that it is difficult for practitioners to interpret and implement the information conveyed to them (Greer, 1988).

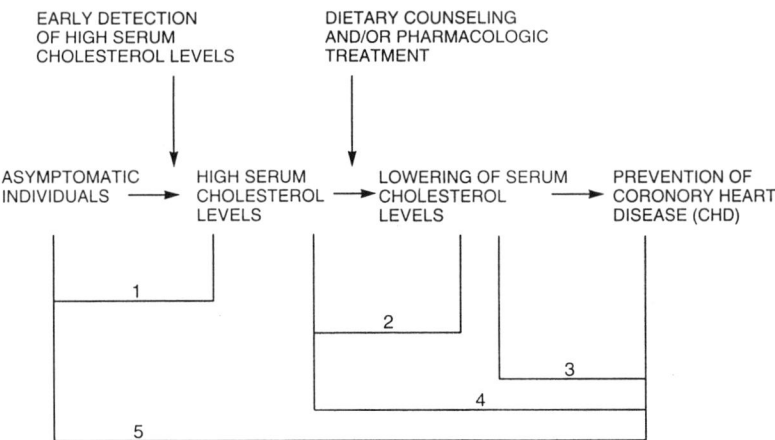

Figure 2.1. Early Detection of High Serum Cholesterol Levels

Source: Battista & Fletcher (1988). Making recommendations on preventive practices: Methodological issues. *American Journal of Preventive Medicine, 4*(4) (suppl. 2), 63. Reprinted with permission.

Another channel is the oral tradition, which is learned in medical school and carried on in the form of continuing medical education activities. Initially organized as fora for scientists to present information to practicing clinicians, these activities are increasingly being performed by practitioners for practitioners. Their impact varies, however, according to different target audiences (Davis, Thomson, Oxman, & Haynes, 1992; Haynes, Davis, McKibbon, & Tugwell, 1984).

Because of the increasing amount of information that the practicing clinician must absorb, the development of clinical practice guidelines is increasingly being perceived as the best possible junction between science and practice and as an instrument for improving quality of care (Battista & Hodge, 1993). Throughout the process, care should be continually monitored so that the initial guidelines can be modified as practice changes and new technologies are developed.

The production of practice guidelines aims at providing practitioners with widely accepted information. The provision of this information, however, must be followed by an array of supporting activities in order to translate into changes of patterns of practice.

The existence of widely accepted information is a necessary but not a sufficient condition for changing practice.

Factors other than knowledge that predispose practitioners to change their practice behavior include skills, judgment, attitudes, and sociodemographic characteristics. For example, important determinants of practice behaviors are the beliefs and attitudes of clinicians with respect to activities with which they would personally comply or that they would offer to their own family members, as well as perceptions of personal efficacy in administering such services (Green, Eriksen, & Schor, 1988). Three sets of factors need to be mobilized in order to change practice behaviors: predisposing, enabling, and reinforcing factors (Green, et al., 1988).

The enabling and reinforcing factors in changing practice behavior are related to the environment in which the clinician practices. Enabling and reinforcing factors are not necessarily different. The timing of their introduction will vary and determine whether they operate as enabling or reinforcing elements. Organizational factors are among the most important enabling and reinforcing factors. Organizational factors influencing the environment include operational tools, practice settings, and financing modalities.

Communication Between Researchers and Policy Makers

Policy makers shape practice environments by allocating resources and introducing regulating mechanisms. Communication of pertinent information to these individuals can thus have an important effect on the shaping of the health care system; however, there are several obstacles to the use of scientific information in public policy. Policy makers interpret research in a context of societal priorities; they are vulnerable to the biases of individual scientists and experts; and their environment predisposes them to accept scientific information that is politically convenient. In addition, the probabilistic nature of scientific information contrasts with a need for certainty in policy making (Hammond, Mumpower, Dennis, Fitch, & Crumpacker, 1983).

The processes of science and those of policy making are fundamentally different (Battista, 1992): The positivist approach of the first can clash with the interpretive process of the latter, which seeks not just one isolated truth at a time but a balance between society's conflicting priorities and values (Lindblom, 1959).

Because of the difficulties of communication, intermediate organizations for the assessment of health care technology have emerged, with the specific purpose of bridging science and policy making. Technology assessment has three distinguishing characteristics. First, its policy orientation sets it apart from health-related research (Banta, Behney, & Willems, 1981, esp. pp. 61-72). This position is not a comfortable one for the assessors, who can easily be accused by scientists of lacking rigor in their methods while being chided by policy makers for lacking relevance. Second, it is not a new discipline; rather, it is both a field and a process of integrating a variety of disciplines as it brings together information on the technical properties, safety, efficacy, effectiveness, and efficiency of interventions and on a variety of other dimensions such as the social consequences and ethical aspects of the introduction of technology (Fuchs & Garber, 1990). Its third distinguishing feature is the variety of methods it uses to synthesize scientific information.

Independent technology assessment bodies have assumed a new role in the flow of information between researchers, policy makers, practitioners, and the media. An example that illustrates this development is taken from the experience of the Conseil d'Evaluation des Technologies de la Santé du Québec (CETS), which performed an evaluation of the routine use of preoperative chest X-ray examinations (PCX) at the request of Quebec's Minister of Health. An internal report of the Ministry (Caron, personal communication, 1991) had documented that the routine use of this procedure totaled an annual cost of $10.6 million.

An analysis of existing data on the 457,000 PCXs requested yearly showed that only 1% of these X rays revealed an unexpected anomaly of the lung, and more importantly, that treatment was modified due to this discovery in only 0.1% of cases (CETS, 1992). The risks of the procedure were shown to outweigh its potential benefits: The CETS estimated that not only did the PCX lead to preoperative delays in the case of false positive results, but the unnecessary exposure to radiation could lead to four mortalities per year for every 400,000 patients.

Despite the limitations of known educational approaches, in this specific case the CETS recommended to the Minister that the data simply be made available to all health care organizations, instead of immediately imposing regulations. A follow-up study will be conducted at the end of 1993 to document changes in the utilization rate of PCX.

Communication With the Media and the Public

Researchers communicate with clinicians in order to convey scientific information and with policy makers in order to help set the agenda for practice, but ultimately, the information they produce is aimed at improving the health of the public. Hence, communication with the public, primarily through the news media, becomes important.

Unfortunately, the priorities of health care professionals and of the news media conflict in several significant ways. In effect, the media aim to entertain as well as to inform; almost all media organizations must exist as profit-making companies; they attempt, for the most part, to reflect society rather than to change it; they cover short-term events rather than long-term campaigns; and they try to deliver salient rather than complex information (Atkin & Arkin, 1990). Because they provide the physical context for communicating information to the public, however, those who wish to send effective messages to a large audience should develop an understanding of the logic of journalism.

The news media can be viewed as a four-tier loom that weaves health messages into a finely crafted fabric: radio offers directness and immediacy; television provides powerful cinematic revelation; daily newspapers flesh out detail and background; and magazines explore issues with perceptions developed over widely spaced deadlines (Atkin & Arkin, 1990).

The media have responded to an increased market for health care reporting by providing more coverage of medical news: at least one fourth of all articles in American daily newspapers are in some way related to health (Atkin & Arkin, 1990). There is a lack of Canadian data on the coverage of medical issues. Despite their power to reach a large audience, journalists operate in a context of several structural constraints, with the main limitations imposed by time, financial considerations, editorial judgments, and audience preferences (Nelkin, 1987). The guiding principle is that of time: News for mass consumption has to be packageable in daily bites, as competition and the daily cycle require it to be shaped into small, salient packages even when the events it describes may not be easily adaptable to that form (Meyer, 1990). The time that can be spent researching and producing news stories and the length of time during which these stories will remain newsworthy are both severely limited.

An understanding of how journalists function also includes recognition of two other constraints: The newsroom demands conflict and the appearance of objectivity. Attempts to balance conflicting claims often reduce news to near binary simplicity: "AIDS is transmitted heterosexually" "No it isn't" (Meyer, 1990, p. 57). Positions that clearly differ are attractive to the journalist because their juxtaposition presents conflict, sharpens the drama, and heightens interest. Yet although most reporters package information in black and white, health care professionals strive for shades of grey in the understanding of complex issues. To the health care research community, uncertainty is often the "central knowable truth" (Klaidman, 1990, p. 67); to journalists, information is most desirable in absolute terms and should be reducible to the categories of good news or bad news. The nightly newscasts present "either promising applications or perilous effects, of triumphant progress or tragic risks" (Nelkin, 1987).

Problematic Crossings

In a perfect world, health care information would flow in a linear fashion. In reality, the transfer of information from one level to the other is disorderly, if not altogether chaotic (players at the different levels of the health care system often disregard the logical flow of information).

An example of the potential hazards of taking communication detours is the storm that occurred in Quebec in 1992 when research results were released directly to the media and the public on PSA (prostate specific antigen), an early detection test for prostate cancer. A group of researchers had published the results of a study aimed at determining the sensitivity and specificity of this new screening procedure in the *Journal of Urology* (Labrie et al., 1992). The study used accepted methodologies and produced important and useful results on the performance of this detection test; however, it did not purport to show that the systematic application of this screening intervention would decrease mortality from prostate cancer in the male population. In the scientific community, this study was treated simply as an additional piece of information to be further integrated in the overall debate about early detection of prostate cancer (Lange, 1992; Stamey, 1992).

Nonetheless, the senior investigator interacted directly with the news media to inform them of the findings. Whether the investigator presented the information in an advantageous fashion or whether the media misjudged the significance of these results is difficult to determine. Although investigators certainly have a stake in creating enthusiasm for such information in order to carry out further research and attract more funding, the media are also keen to unveil a miracle detection intervention. In any event, the public's interpretation of the message was that prostate cancer could now be cured if detected early and that this test should be implemented in a province-wide early detection program as soon as possible. Very soon, hospital administrators were receiving phone calls from patients requesting this new test. One journalist forcefully denounced the actions of the investigator, turning the issue into a political debate (Dufresne, 1992). Putting the facts in their proper context required the mobilization of several players in the health care system.

Conclusion

Although the existing communication networks among researchers, policy makers, practitioners, the media, and the public can transform knowledge into better care, there are several ways that the process of disseminating scientific information can break down.

Many new questions need to be dealt with. Do the differences in the approaches and interests of these different players complement each other or are they irreconcilable? Are there better ways for researchers to create enthusiasm for medical research? Is there a need for an intermediary body to bridge the domains of scientists, policy makers, and the public? How can health care messages be communicated more effectively through the media to the public?

We need to develop a better understanding of the specific contribution of each level of communication and to establish links between these levels in order to avoid careless exchanges that could become counterproductive to the ultimate objective of making rational choices in our health care system.

References

Atkin, C., & Arkin, E. B. (1990). Issues and initiatives in communicating health information to the public. In C. Atkin & L. Wallack (Eds.), *Mass communication and public health* (pp. 13-40). Newbury Park, CA: Sage.

Banta, H. D., Behney, C. J., & Willems, J. A. (1981). *Toward rational technology in medicine: Considerations for health policy.* New York: Springer-Verlag.

Battista, R. N. (1992). Health care technology assessment: Linking science and policy-making. *Canadian Medical Association Journal, 146*(4), 461-462.

Battista, R. N., Contandriopoulos, A. P., Champagne, F., Williams, J. I., Pineault, R., & Boyle, P. (1989). An integrative framework for health-related research. *Journal of Clinical Epidemiology, 42*(12), 1155-1160.

Battista, R. N., & Fletcher, S. W. (1988). Making recommendations on preventive practices: Methodological issues. *American Journal of Preventive Medicine, 4*(4, Suppl.), 53-67.

Battista, R. N., & Hodge, M. J. (1993). Clinical practice guidelines: Between science and art. *Canadian Medical Association Journal, 148*(3), 385-389.

Becher, T. (1989). Patterns of communication. In *Academic tribes and territories: Intellectual enquiry and the cultures of disciplines.* Philadelphia: Open University Press.

Canadian Task Force on the Periodic Health Examination. (1979). The periodic health examination. *Canadian Medical Association Journal, 121*, 1193-1254.

Conseil d'Evaluation des Technologies de la Santé du Québec. (1992). *Routine preoperative chest X rays.* Montreal: CETS.

Davis, D. A., Thomson, M. A., Oxman, A. D., & Haynes, R. B. (1992). Evidence for the effectiveness of CME: A review of 50 randomized controlled trials. *Journal of the American Medical Association, 268*(9), 1111-1117.

Dufresne, J. (1992, April 25). La saga de la prostate. *La Presse,* p. B3.

Fuchs, V. R., & Garber, A. M. (1990). The new technology assessment. *New England Journal of Medicine, 324*,(10), 673-677.

Green, L. W., Eriksen, M. P., & Schor, E. L. (1988). Preventive practices by physicians: Behavioral determinants and potential interventions. *American Journal of Preventive Medicine, 4*(4, Suppl.), 101-107.

Greer, A. L. (1988). The state of the art versus the state of the science: The diffusion of new medical technologies into practice. *International Journal of Technology Assessment in Health Care, 4*, 5-26.

Haltery, L. H. (1986). Interdisciplinary research management. In D. E. Chubin, A. L. Porter, F. A. Rossini, & T. Connolly (Eds.), *Interdisciplinary analysis and research* (pp. 13-28). Mount Airy, MD: Lomond Publications.

Hammond, K. R., Mumpower, J., Dennis, R. L., Fitch, S., & Crumpacker, W. (1983). Fundamental obstacles to the use of scientific information in public policy making. *Technological Forecasting and Social Change, 24,* 287-297.

Haynes, R. B., Davis, D. A., McKibbon, A., & Tugwell, P. (1984). A critical appraisal of the efficacy of continuing medical education. *Journal of the American Medical Association, 251*(1), 61-64.

Klaidman, S. (1990). Roles and responsibilities of journalists. In C. Atkin & L. Wallack (Eds.), *Mass communication and public health* (pp. 60-70). Newbury Park, CA: Sage.

Klein, J. T. (1990). *Interdisciplinarity: History, theory, and practice.* Detroit: Wayne State University Press.

Kuhn, J. T. (1970). *The structure of scientific revolutions* (2nd ed.). Chicago: University of Chicago Press.

Labrie, F., Dupont, A., Suburu, R., Cusan, L., Tremblay, M., Gomez, J.-L., & Emond, J. (1992). Serum prostate specific antigen as a pre-screening test for prostate cancer. *Journal of Urology, 147,* 846-852.

Lange, P. H. (1992). Editorial comment. *Journal of Urology, 147,* 852.

Lindblom, C. E. (1959). The science of muddling through. *Public Administration Review, 19*(Spring), 79-88.

Luszki, M. B. (1958). *Interteam research methods and problems* (chap. 6, pp. 137-169). New York: New York University Press.

MacDonald, W. R. (1986). Characteristics of interdisciplinary research teams. In D. E. Chubin, A. L. Porter, F. A. Rossini, & T. Connolly (Eds.), *Interdisciplinary analysis and research* (pp. 395-406). Mount Airy, MD: Lomond Publications.

McGlynn, E. A., Kosecoff, J., & Brook, R. H. (1990). Format and conduct of consensus development conferences—Multination comparison. *International Journal of Technology Assessment in Health Care, 6,* 450-469.

Meyer, P. (1990). News media responsiveness to public health. In C. Atkin & L. Wallack (Eds.), *Mass communication and public health* (pp. 52-59). Newbury Park, CA: Sage.

Nelkin, D. (1987). *Selling science: How the press covers science and technology.* New York: Freeman.

Stamey T. A. (1992). [Editorial comment.] *Journal of Urology, 147,* 851-852.

U.S. Preventive Services Task Force. (1989). *Guide to clinical preventive services.* Baltimore, MD: Williams & Wilkins.

Woolf, S. H., Battista, R. N., Anderson, G. M., Logan, A. G., Wang, E., & the Canadian Task Force on the Periodic Health Examination. (1990). Assessing the clinical effectiveness of preventive maneuvers: Analytic principles and systematic methods in reviewing evidence and developing clinical practice recommendations. *Journal of Clinical Epidemiology, 43*(9), 891-905.

3 Toward an Ethic in Dissemination of New Knowledge in Primary Care Research

ERIC M. MESLIN

In the rich literature on the ethics of research (Katz, 1972; Levine, 1986; Veatch, 1987), discussions of the ethical issues that arise in the dissemination of new knowledge have not occupied much space. Instead, attention has largely centered on "topical" issues, such as informed consent, risk-benefit assessments, and the use of placebo controls—that is, those issues that arise at the point of designing and conducting studies. Perhaps this is because these are the points at which interventions occur and over which regulations exist (Levine, 1986), and perhaps it is because of the concern with cases of fraudulent data gathering or presentation (Kohn, 1988; Miller & Hersen, 1992). What both explanations have in common, however, is their emphasis on the ethical issues that arise in attempting to prevent harm to patients, rather than on the positive, aspirational components of the system of values that ought to inform the dissemination of new knowledge. Such a system of values, centering on the ethical issues that confront primary care researchers, is the focus of this chapter.

Philosophers have long been occupied with questions about knowledge, such as how one *knows* things such as places, people, or truths—the study of epistemology. The standard analysis of

AUTHOR'S NOTE: Research for this manuscript was partially sponsored by a grant from the Social Sciences and Humanities Research Council of Canada (#806-91-0002).

knowledge, which dates from Plato, is that knowledge is equivalent to "true belief with an account," where an account would show why what is believed must be so (O'Connor, 1982). In its more modern form (and one more relevant to scientific investigation), *knowledge* is defined as "justified true belief" where the believer has "adequate evidence" (Chisholm, 1957). The details of the philosophic debates need not be recapitulated here, except to suggest that any philosophic analysis of the theory of knowledge recognizes that there may be several kinds of knowledge, with the most common distinction being that between propositional knowledge ("knowing that") and instrumental knowledge ("knowing how"). Of course, scientific knowledge falls into both categories; but as the theme of this volume attests, the value in disseminating new knowledge from primary care research is not only that a better understanding of medical problems will be available (e.g., knowing *that* a pragmatic asthma morbidity index can be derived from a patient questionnaire; Jones, Chapter 4 this volume), but that there is a specific value in disseminating knowledge where it has the potential to change practitioner behavior (e.g., knowing *how* to integrate research findings through evidence-based family medicine; Elmslie, Chapter 13 this volume).

Understanding the difference between propositional and instrumental knowledge is only the first step in recognizing the ethical issues that arise in disseminating new knowledge. Other terms need to be defined. I will assume a broad, general definition of *disseminate*, as found in the *Webster's Third New International Dictionary:* "to spread or send out freely or widely . . . make widespread." In contrast, I will restrict the use of "new knowledge" to a more manageable distinction between "data" and "information," which are related terms. By *data*, I am referring to raw data, the products of research, be they the mathematical calculations or findings of a quantitative intervention (e.g., the number count of patients who responded to a therapy, or the percentage of tumor reduction achieved by chemotherapy), or the experiential findings of qualitative research (e.g., the descriptions that families give of how they cope with loss). By *information* I am referring to the first (or next) product of data organization or analysis. This includes the organization or presentation of data (whether it be in tables or narratives). Although this distinction will not be rigidly adhered to ("medical information" is one way of referring to different taxonomic categorizations of data; Feinstein, 1987), it is important to bear in mind the difference between the specific products of research that may be disseminated or shared, and the form that the information itself takes. It is already well known, for example, that the way information is presented or "framed" affects how it is received and understood (Tversky & Kahneman, 1984).

This chapter is divided into four parts, which taken together could provide the basis for the development of an ethic of dissemination. By *ethic*, I am referring to a description of a set of values of a practice or activity; and I say "the basis for an ethic" because the description of a full philosophical justification is beyond the scope of this chapter.

The first part describes the elements of the broad *scientific ethic*. The second part describes the components of a *human research ethic*. This ethic is a narrower version of a more general ethic of scientific investigation and includes issues that arise from the conception, design, and conduct of research involving human subjects. The third part extends the second by examining the *publication ethic*, looking at the narrowness of many of the rules and expectations about publication. And the fourth part suggests that the above ethics do not alone capture all the issues that arise in the context of dissemination of new knowledge and addresses these remaining issues in a discussion of a unique *dissemination ethic*.

The Scientific Ethic

Investigators, whether they work in basic or applied research, have been informed through a variety of sources of a set of expectations regarding the conduct of their research. This general set of values can be called a *"scientific ethic."* Although it is beyond the scope of this chapter to illuminate the features of the scientific ethic (that being a task for the philosophy of science), there is considerable discussion about the presumption that science is a value-free enterprise whose goal is seeking truth (Merton, 1957).

Differing views have emerged regarding the advisability of even presuming that objectivity is a worthy approach to take in assessing actions or decisions of others (Carse, 1991; Savan, 1988). Even more pointedly, Longino (1990) has observed that even though it is nonsense to suggest that science is value-free, it has two very different types of values. *Constitutive* values are governing rules that allow researchers to pursue the general goal of scientific enquiry, which she takes to be "the production of explanations of the natural world" (Longino, 1990, p. 4). These values describe what counts as acceptable scientific practice or method; for example, "the satisfaction of such criteria as truth, accuracy, simplicity, predictability and breadth" (p. 4). *Contextual* values are "personal, social and cultural values, those group or individual preferences about what ought to be" (p. 4). I share Longino's view that these two types of values are inseparable in science. Moreover, a scientific ethic ought explicitly to acknowledge the inseparable link between scientific values (even objectivity has a normative foundation), and those ethical values about what should be investigated; between the mere description of results, and the influence of personal and contextual values on the activity of dissemination.

The Human Research Ethic

The *"human research ethic"* can be understood as a more specific version of this broader scientific ethic. If the scientific ethic explains the moral foundation for what Longino (1990, p. 4) calls "explanations of the natural world," the human research ethic provides the justification for the conduct of research involving human subjects. Among the values that inform this ethic are the following: (a) all research involving human subjects must be reviewed prospectively by an institutional review board (in Canada these are known as Research Ethics Boards, or REBs); (b) research that is not scientifically valid cannot be considered ethical, because flawed designs would expose research subjects to unnecessary risk (Parkin, 1993); and (c) subjects/participants must be protected from the risks of harm that might occur in research—principally through their ability to give informed consent to participate, or if this is not possible, through the ability of a surrogate or proxy to provide this permission (Medical Research Council of Canada [MRC], 1987). Additional elements of the human research ethic that pertain to vulnerable populations and to special categories of research have been described (U.S. National Commission, 1978; Veatch, 1987).

These expectations arose as a direct response to the revelations of the tragic examples of "research" undertaken during World War II, and were initially described in the Nuremberg Code (Annas & Grodin, 1992; Rothman, 1991). They have been more comprehensively described in existing guidelines and regulations for research on human subjects (Council of International Organizations of Medical Societies [CIOMS], 1982; MRC, 1987; U.S. Federal Policy, 1991; World Medical Association, 1975), and continue to hold moral force. The human research ethic reflects a 15-year-old paradigm, one that was articulated by the U.S. National Commission for the Protection of Human Subjects in the *Belmont Report* (1978) in response to reports of research abuse in the United States (Beecher, 1966; Katz, 1972). This paradigm envisioned the role of researchers as one of seeking knowledge and the role of institutional review boards as one of protecting human subjects against specified (typically physical) harms. According to this paradigm, protocols (usually placebo-controlled randomized clinical trials) are reviewed prospectively by these committees, which make their judgments about the merit of studies and the protection of subjects, trusting investigators to carry out the study as described.

There is much to recommend such a paradigm. It can be used for quality assurance, setting professional standards, and suggesting a method for assuring consistency in the process of review. It has been valuable for sensitizing researchers to the ethical principles and guidelines for conducting research, and perhaps even for teaching young investigators about the minimal requirements for obtaining ethics approval prior to (or in conjunction with) submission to external peer review agencies for funding (Meslin, 1993). Ethical principles of *respect for autonomy, beneficence, nonmaleficence,* and *justice* provide the philosophic foundation for the evaluation of research (Beauchamp & Childress, 1989).

What this research ethic paradigm must face, however, are a number of new and in many ways more prevalent issues confronting researchers (Veatch, 1987). For example, it still cannot ensure that investigators will have the type of character traits to ensure that ethically acceptable behavior occurs; something that Beecher (1966) believed was a research subject's best protection against harm. This may be because a "virtuous disposition" is best learned by observing such behavior in others, and few of the curricula in

North American medical science programs explicitly deal with the subject of research ethics.

The paradigm also has not attended to the problems that arise when physicians act as both caregivers and investigators (Schafer, 1982), a problem that could be particularly acute with primary care physicians. Nor does it address the phenomenon (increasingly evident in oncology and AIDS research) of patients actively seeking enrollment in clinical trials, believing them to be the best chance of therapy (Till, Sutherland, & Meslin, 1992). The existing guidelines are being stretched somewhat in recent requirements to permit REBs to inquire of investigators about their financial arrangements for conducting research (College of Physicians and Surgeons of Ontario [CPSO], 1992), and in its ability to evaluate new methods of research, such as prospective development of large data sets as found in larger clinical epidemiology studies (Squires, 1992) or some types of qualitative research. Finally, it does not articulate the expectations regarding publication and dissemination. These, as discussed below, have evolved separately.

The Publication Ethic

Scientific information is the currency in which researchers and practitioners conduct their business, and those who have more, better, more current, and more convincing data are the richer. Related to this, the *publication ethic* may best be described as a set of expectations about the proper method for preparing and presenting data and information within the literature.

If the human research ethic is a narrower version of the scientific ethic, so too is the publication ethic a portion of the broader set of expectations that apply to research. Its assumptions include the following: (a) science is a self-correcting activity in which falsity and error will be rooted out through the quality control function of peer review and journal publication; (b) it is preferable to publish positive research findings, because they advance knowledge; and (c) although information ought to be published for its own sake, the purpose of publishing one's research is to facilitate the goals of science generally. (For the basic scientist, this includes an explanation of how the world works; for the clinical investigator, it includes the expectation that information will advance knowledge about the treatment of disease and illness in human beings.) Journal editors have added further elements to this ethic, including: (d) a requirement that research that reports the results of studies involving human subjects should conform to the principles of the Declaration of Helsinki and be approved by the investigator's REB (International Committee of Medical Journal Editors [ICMJE], 1991); and (e) research findings should be published in the peer-reviewed literature for one's peers prior to general release to the public—the so-called Ingelfinger Rule.

Regrettably, it has become evident that these expectations are not always met. Peer review does not always find error and indeed may have its own problems (Longino, 1990; Peters & Ceci, 1982). The well-known reality (rarely defended in the open literature) is the oft-cited "publish or perish" rule (Brackbill & Hellegers, 1980), an expectation placed on researchers—especially young ones—that professional advancement is measured in the number of publications rather than their quality. Although there is some evidence that this expectation is abating (Harvard University has altered its rank and tenure requirements to focus on quality of publications rather than quantity), it has been suggested that a different expectation has emerged: there still appears to be preferential bias among journal editors to publish only positive findings, not negative or disconfirming ones (Weisse, 1986).

Compared to the research ethic, the historical sources for the publication ethic are more difficult to trace, but it is likely that its expectations and guidelines emerged from the numerous cases of research fraud and misconduct reported in the literature (Broad & Wade, 1982; Kohn, 1988; Lowy & Meslin, 1993; Miller & Hersen, 1992), and from more recent concerns about conflict of interest, particularly in the control of industry-sponsored research (Porter & Malone, 1992). The elements of the narrow publication ethic are now being collected in both general guidelines and specific authorship guidelines (Huth, 1986). Like the human research ethic, a set of principles has emerged for authorship relating to the type and amount of participation that any one person must have in order to be listed as a coauthor. For example, these principles would exclude from consideration as authors those persons whose sole contribution was data collection.

Although these principles have emerged from a larger set of guidelines that describe the format of journal submissions (ICMJE,

1991), they have not resolved all publication issues. It is still the case that junior investigators are either required or even coerced into including more senior investigators (such as the head of a team or lab) on multiply authored papers, even when the senior authors did not participate in any aspect of the study. Similarly, although the ICMJE Guidelines require an assurance that studies involving human subjects have been conducted in accordance with the standards of an institutional Research Ethics Board, this assurance still requires some degree of trust. Likewise, even though manuscripts should "describe statistical methods with enough detail to enable a knowledgeable reader with access to the original data to verify the results" (ICMJE, 1991, p. 425), the sheer number of journal submissions makes the policing of this requirement somewhat difficult to imagine. Finally, the publication ethic may actually conflict with a more patient-centered ethic that encourages rapid dissemination of findings in order to affect practitioner behavior.

Toward a Dissemination Ethic
for Primary Care Research

In the previous three sections, I have suggested that the foundation for an ethic of dissemination has been laid by a broader scientific ethic, a human research ethic, and a publication ethic. Is its set of expectations and values sufficiently different from these other ethics to warrant separate treatment? I suggest here that although there is some overlap, the elements of a dissemination ethic are unique enough to be considered separately.

Two initial distinctions can be drawn. With regard to the human research ethic, the focus is on the conduct of an investigation, with the principal concerns being the scientific quality of the study and the acceptability of involving human beings in an activity that is not primarily intended to benefit them; in contrast, the primary concerns of the dissemination ethic relate to the management of the results (both data and information) obtained and to the intended impact of the knowledge on clinicians. With regard to the publication ethic, the concern is with the creation and presentation of information in a manner suitable for scientific and clinical consumption through the medium of journals; in contrast, the dissemination ethic is concerned with the method by which knowledge is transmitted to those who will make use of it, irrespective of whether the information is presented in published form in a peer-reviewed journal or a regular circulation newspaper. Because dissemination can occur through print, audio, or visual media, there is nothing that prima facie precludes on ethical grounds the dissemination of information to clinicians in whatever form it might take. This is because its ethical justification is based jointly on a scientific ethic and a therapeutic one: Without new information, knowledge will not advance; without getting it into the hands of clinicians who can use it, the information will have no benefit to patients.

An ethic of dissemination ought to make reference to the importance of sharing research information in order to effect a positive change in clinical practice. The idea that one ought to share research data is not a new concept, the benefits having already been discussed by the U.S. National Academy of Sciences (Fienberg, Martin, & Straf, 1985). Sharing data permits scientists to collaborate, to attempt replication of study results, and to participate in activities where synergistically the knowledge created is greater than the sum of its parts. The justification for sharing data is straightforward: for research that is conducted with monies from the public purse, public responsibility alone requires the dissemination of the knowledge obtained from that support. (To say that publicly funded researchers are "accountable" to the public is only partially correct: because there is no specific relationship between the public and the researcher, the public does not carry any authority; however, if "accountable" means "able to give an account of," certainly researchers should be held accountable, both to explain how monies were spent and what the money actually paid for.) It is more reasonable to hold researchers "responsible" to the public in that they should be "able to respond" to requests for information about what public monies paid for. Even for research funded through private sources, the obligation to disseminate findings per se remains. Although additional constraints on prior release of data for proprietary reasons (e.g., patent rights) may place some limits on the timing of dissemination, practitioner behavior cannot be influenced without the availability of the knowledge. Therefore, it is in the sponsor's best interest to ensure prompt dissemination.

What has not been discussed extensively, however, is the concept of sharing knowledge (by dissemination) for the express purpose of changing practitioner behavior and positively affecting patient care. For example, rarely is a full research protocol published in the literature, which would provide a complete and accurate account of the scientific value of the research, in addition to its validity (Freedman, 1987). Reading a final report of a study (albeit, one that includes a discussion of the background, methods, results, and limitations) does not provide the scientific community with a complete account of it from conception to conduct to analysis. Similarly, I suspect that rarely do research subjects actively seek out the data itself, preferring (if they have an interest) in learning (a) whether the intervention being tested had a favorable result, and (b) whether they received the beneficial intervention, if they were randomized.

Many individuals and groups are involved in developing new knowledge, preparing it for publication and dissemination, funding or otherwise supporting it, and having an interest in it. A consensus statement regarding the responsibility to disseminate new knowledge by researchers, academics, editors, professional bodies, and others appears in Chapter 7 of this volume, so I will not duplicate the points made there. Rather, I will highlight one specific dissemination relationship that has not been fully appreciated.

Few mechanisms exist for imparting a dissemination ethic, particularly to patients. In part, as I have suggested above, it is not clear who might bear this responsibility, given that many have a partial responsibility to disseminate some form of new knowledge, and many have (or believe that they have) a right to receive it. But little attention has been given to the best strategies for ensuring that patients as subjects, or even future patients, are part of the loop. Journal editors certainly bear some responsibility for ensuring that scientifically meritorious and ethically acceptable research be published (i.e., factually correct information printed in a journal), but this is not identical to disseminating, and it certainly is not targeted at patients. Similarly, institutional review committees bear some responsibility even if in only the most tangential ways: In assuring that research is scientifically and ethically acceptable, approval can be provided on request to journal editors who are increasingly requiring such approval letters when considering publication. In the future, by receiving data monitoring and safety reports, the review committee will be in a position to suspend or stop ongoing research if convinced that it is too dangerous to be completed or if the benefits are overwhelming. This will have the net effect of accelerating dissemination of the results to the scientific community, if only to report premature termination of a study. By requiring that consent forms disclose the fact that a report of the study may be made available to subjects upon completion of the study, patients will have access to study information. These measures are modest, however. Carol Herbert devotes more to this issue in Chapter 10 of this volume.

References

Annas, G. J., & Grodin, M. A. (1992). *The Nazi doctors and the Nuremberg Code: Human rights in human experimentation.* New York: Oxford University Press.

Beauchamp, T. L., & Childress, J. F. (1989). *Principles of medical ethics* (3rd ed.). New York: Oxford University Press.

Beecher, H. K. (1966). Ethics and clinical research. *New England Journal of Medicine, 274*(4), 1354-1360.

Brackbill, Y., & Hellegers, A. E. (1980). Ethics and editors. *Hastings Center Report, 10,* 20-22.

Broad, W., & Wade, N. (1982). *Betrayers of the truth: Fraud and deceit in the halls of science.* New York: Simon & Schuster.

Carse, L. L. (1991). The "voice of care": Implications for bioethical education. *Journal of Medicine and Philosophy, 16,* 5-28.

Chisholm, R. M. (1957). *Perceiving: A philosophical study.* Ithaca, NY: Cornell University Press.

College of Physicians and Surgeons of Ontario. (1992, August). Physicians and the pharmaceutical industry. *College Notices, No. 26.*

Council of International Organizations of Medical Societies. (1982). *Proposed international guidelines for research on human subjects.* Geneva: Author.

Feinstein, A. R. (1987). *Clinimetrics.* New Haven, CT: Yale University Press.

Fienberg, S. E., Martin, M. E., & Straf, M. L. (Eds.). (1985). *Sharing research data.* Washington, DC: National Academy Press.

Freedman, B. (1987). Scientific value and validity as ethical requirements for research: A proposed explication. *IRB: A Review of Human Subjects Research, 9,* 7-10.

Huth, E. J. (1986). Guidelines on authorship of medical papers. *Annals of Internal Medicine, 104,* 269-274.

International Committee of Medical Journal Editors [ICMJE]. (1991). Uniform requirements for manuscripts submitted to biomedical journals. *New England Journal of Medicine, 324,* 424-428.

Katz, J. (1972). *Experimentation on human beings.* New York: Russell Sage.

Kohn, A. (1988). *False prophets: Fraud and error in science and medicine*. Oxford: Basil Blackwell.

Levine, R. J. (1986). *Ethics and regulation of clinical research*. New Haven, CT: Yale University Press.

Longino, H. E. (1990). *Science as social knowledge*. Princeton, NJ: Princeton University Press.

Lowy, F. H., & Meslin, E. M. (1993). Fraud in medical research. In G. Koren (Ed.), *Ethics in pediatric research* (pp. 293-307). Malabar, FL: Kreiger.

Medical Research Council of Canada. (1987). *Guidelines on research involving human subjects*. Ottawa: Ministry of Supply and Services.

Merton, R. K. (1957). Priorities in scientific discovery: A chapter in the sociology of science. *American Sociological Review, 22*, 635-651.

Meslin, E. M. (1993). Ethical issues in the substantive and procedural aspects of research ethics review. *Health Law in Canada, 13*, 179-191.

Miller, D. J., & Hersen, M. (1992). Misconduct and fraud in the empirical sciences: History and review. In D. J. Miller & M. Hersen (Eds.), *Research fraud in the behavioral and biomedical sciences* (pp. 3-16). New York: John Wiley.

O'Connor, D. J. (1982). *Introduction to the theory of knowledge*. Minneapolis: University of Minnesota Press.

Parkin, P. (1993). The relationship between ethics and science in pediatric research. In G. Koren (Ed.), *Ethics in pediatric research* (pp. 221-234). Malabar, FL: Kreiger.

Peters, D., & Ceci, S. (1982). Peer review practices of psychological journals: The fate of published articles submitted again. *Behavioral and Brain Sciences, 5*, 187-195.

Porter, R. J., & Malone, T. E. (Eds.). (1992). *Biomedical research: Collaboration and conflict of interest*. Baltimore, MD: Johns Hopkins University Press.

Rothman, D. J. (1991). *Strangers at the bedside: A history of how law and bioethics transformed medical decision making*. New York: Basic Books.

Savan, B. (1988). *Science under siege: The myth of objectivity in scientific research*. Toronto: Canadian Broadcasting Corporation.

Schafer, A. (1982). The ethics of the randomized clinical trial. *New England Journal of Medicine, 307*, 719-724.

Squires, B. (1992). Confidentiality and research. *Canadian Medical Association Journal, 147*(9), 1229.

Till, J. E., Sutherland, H. J., & Meslin, E. M. (1992). Is there a role for preference assessments in research on quality of life in oncology? *Quality of Life Research, 1*, 31-40.

Tversky, A., & Kahneman, D. (1984). Choices, values, and frames. *American Psychologist, 39*, 341-350.

U.S. Federal Policy for Protection of Human Subjects. (1991). 86 Code of Federal Regulations 28004.

U.S. National Commission for the Protection of Human Subjects of Biomedical and Behavioral Research. (1978). *Belmont report: Ethical principles and guidelines for protection of human subjects of research*. Washington, DC: Department of Health and Human Services.

Veatch, R. M. (1987). *The patient as partner*. Bloomington: Indiana University Press.

Weisse, A. B. (1986, March). Say it isn't so: Positive thinking and the publication of medical research. *Hospital Practice*, pp. 23-25.

World Medical Association. (1964). Declaration of Helsinki (revised 1975, 1983, 1989). In T. L. Beauchamp & L. Walters (Eds.), *Contemporary issues in bioethics* (3rd ed.) (pp. 421-423). Belmont, CA: Wadsworth.

4 Disseminating New Knowledge to Other Researchers

ROGER JONES

Special problems surround the dissemination of new knowledge gained in primary health care research, and it is perhaps worth reflecting on some of these. Primary health care incorporates the work of many professional groups, including family physicians and general practitioners, nurses, epidemiologists, health economists, and social scientists; all of whom may be engaged, often in teams, on research activities. This implies a variety and complexity of research output demanding different formats of presentation and communication in a variety of settings (Haynes, 1990). (For example, clinical research undertaken in general practice may have important messages to send across the interface between primary and secondary care for the provision of hospital services; similarly, the work of health economists and family practice researchers may generate information of importance to health care planners and administrators.) Primary care research is also frequently opportunistic and sometimes sporadic, not least because its tradition and culture are still in the developmental stages. Looking beyond North America and Europe, it is clear that special difficulties arise in the communication of research work across social, economic, and political interfaces.

At a deeper level, primary health care itself is responsive to the constantly changing social, economic, and physical environments in any given national or local setting. Thus similar questions may need to be reexamined when issues of funding, resourcing, models of health care delivery, or social expectations shift and change. Although capable of leading-edge research, primary care must also necessarily be responsive to developments in biomedicine and to the application and evaluation of new technologies. Accordingly, research in this field is generally nonlinear, in contradistinction to much of the traditional research activity of biomedicine, where progress is linear and incremental and small steps are made along a frequently predetermined pathway (McWhinney, 1991). Vulnerability to changes caused by all these extraneous factors can lead to difficulties in sustaining program activity in a defined research area.

Research in primary care remains a minority activity: unnecessary in crude career terms for professionals working outside academic institutions; frequently driven by individual enthusiasms and preoccupations; and often highly site-specific and not necessarily capable of generalization to other health care delivery systems or settings. Difficulties in obtaining adequate resources for research follow from some of these features, and are felt particularly sharply by practice-based researchers who do not have access to a critical mass of colleagues or to the motivation, support, and expertise found in academic groupings. Nonetheless, there is ample demonstration that individual researchers are capable of making substantial contributions. The next section considers some ways to incorporate their enthusiasms, skills, and achievements.

Finding Other Researchers

The primary care research community is diverse and scattered, which can make current and unpublished activities difficult to discern. Although the literature review that precedes any research project will indicate the extent of published work in the area of interest, keeping abreast of the literature is difficult and in any case is likely to be a poor substitute for direct contact with other workers with shared interests. Frequently the only way to validate research questions, gain support for their intrinsic interest and merit, confirm the appropriateness of the methodologies to be employed, and determine the likely significance of the information gained is through peer group discussion and participation in research meetings and conferences. For researchers working outside university departments, such interaction may be particularly important, but is also likely to be difficult to achieve. Both local and national groups exist and can help in many ways.

LOCAL AND REGIONAL GROUPS

In the United Kingdom, groups have sprung up across the country where new entrants to general practice who share enthusiasms for practice development, audit, and research can gather informally, often with co-opted expertise from academic departments. The common factors in these departments tend to include inexperience and uncertainty, which, when recognized, can be turned to advantage and provide the bases for progress and achievement.

A particularly effective support group for young primary care researchers operated in the south of England for several years. This "small r" informally constituted group consisted of a mixture of general practitioners from academic units and National Health Services (NHS) practice, and met about every 3 months in either London, Oxford, or Southampton. Key ingredients that contributed to its success included friendship (we actually liked seeing each other!), openness about doubts about our own work and that of others, acceptance of critical comment, validation and praise for good work, and—perhaps most important of all—that incredible energy that is associated with the excitement of setting out in research and with being under the age of 35.

Regional research groups that draw membership from several towns or cities have also proved successful, with a key ingredient being input from academic units including university departments of general practice, epidemiology, and medical statistics. Examples include the Cumbrian research group in the Lake District of northern England, and the Georgian research group, centered in Winchester in the south of England. Few of these initiatives have, however, led to the development of an enduring structure such as the Ambulatory Sentinel Practice Network (ASPN) in North America. The closest British analogue is the Medical Research Council General Practice Research Framework, a network of more than 200 practices nationwide. This group, though, is more concerned with the collection of high-quality data from primary care than with the initiation of research studies by the practitioners themselves.

NATIONAL GROUPS AND ORGANIZATIONS

The General Practice Research Club was set up in 1969, following an innovative course in research methods organized by the Royal College of General Practitioners. The club has been active for the past 20 years, providing a setting in which general practitioners can meet in a friendly and supportive atmosphere that is also constructively critical. An analysis of nine Club meetings held between 1984 and 1989 (Jones, Wilmot, & Fry, 1991) showed that there were 57 presentations and 2 workshop sessions, 40 of which were original research papers, principally on clinical topics (prevention and health promotion, consultation, workload, and delivery of care). Presenters were asked in a questionnaire survey about how making these presentations impacted on their work. In 11 of the 40 projects, respondents said that significant or very important modification resulted from the presentation and subsequent discussion, and a further 16 reported minor changes. Of 37 presentations reporting preliminary results, research ideas, or unpublished data, 17 led to publication. When asked about the global value of making the presentation, those who were presenting ideas for research rated the experience highest.

The European General Practice Research Workshop is a similar organization providing support for practice-based researchers from many European countries (Jones, 1991).

The contribution of university departments of general practice, which have come into their own during the past decade, has probably been the most important ingredient in the development of a primary care research culture in the United Kingdom. Critical mass, increasing expertise in obtaining research funding and acceptance by the "traditional" research community, coupled with an increasing awareness of the importance of community-based teaching and research and development, have all contributed to their success, which has recently been underpinned by substantially improved central funding from the Department of Health (but not from the Universities Funding Council). This means that the departments are now in a better position to think about a career structure for their staff, nonclinical as well as clinical, and to become less dependent on the generation of income from clinical care activities.

The Association of University Departments of General Practice (AUDGP) is the U.K. analogue of the North American Primary Care Research Group in terms of size, content, and perhaps to a lesser extent membership (which is more similar to that of the Society of Teachers of Family Medicine). Its annual scientific meeting is the most important primary care research conference in the British calendar and is a key opportunity for informal networking as well as formal presentation.

The Royal College of General Practitioners has also, over a similar period, attempted to develop a research strategy for primary care. Important components of its work have been the provision of protected time for NHS general practitioners and of small grant funding. The College has been responsible for a number of initiatives, including the first research methods course, support for the GP Research Club, establishment of the Scientific Foundation Board to provide research grant support, establishment of Research Training Fellowships, start-up funding for the journal *Family Practice,* and, most recently, an experimental Regional Research Fellowship that has had an immense impact on the perceptions and practice of research in the northern region of England.

Two important recent developments have further strengthened the research community in the United Kingdom. One is the increasing interaction between primary care and secondary care researchers, across the interface between community-based and hospital medicine. Important issues such as outpatient referral, hospital admission, and the development of management guidelines by consensus between generalists and specialists have ensured that much clinical and health services research includes a major input from the primary care sector. The second is the formalization of a Department of Health Research and Development strategy, in which the importance of primary care as a key setting for clinical and health services research is explicitly recognized (Peckham, 1991). The NHS's Central Research and Development Committee (CRDC), which is responsible for setting priorities in health care research, has developed a Research and Development (R&D) strategy ensuring that 1.5% of NHS revenues are used for R&D and is coordinating the management of this research activity.

A series of NHS review groups have been established to derive, from expert opinion and wide consultation, a set of research priorities in broad areas including coronary heart disease, stroke, mental illness, physical and complex disabilities, the primary care/secondary care interface, and new technologies. These priorities become the basis for research grant applications and commissioned research at national and regional levels; many of them have significant primary care components. This process will have major implications for the conduct and dissemination of the results of primary care research, and will undoubtedly concentrate minds on the links between research funding, research findings, and changes in professional behavior. These developments are also likely to contribute to a much better understanding of primary care research by other funding bodies and by health services administrators.

Dissemination of Findings

The important and exciting changes in primary care research described above have implications for a parallel enhancement of the opportunities both for doing research and for communicating its results. It could be argued, however, that they have not been accompanied by increasing opportunities for publication of primary care research in peer-reviewed journals. The experience of editors of national and international journals, all of which receive much more than they can publish, suggests that significant difficulties are still being experienced by authors in getting good-quality primary care research into print. Publication decisions can be very difficult when considering issues of generalizability, particularly across social, national, and even regional boundaries because of the essential site-specificity of some primary care research. Research workers in countries with emergent health care systems and poor local dissemination and publication infrastructures often experience great difficulty in getting their work into print.

As the editor of an international primary care journal, *Family Practice,* as well as a researcher and author, I am keenly aware of both the problems of, and opportunities for, dissemination of research work (Jones, 1990). Between 1984 and 1990, 253 original articles were published in *Family Practice*; 33% were from the United Kingdom, 19% from North America, 12% from Scandinavia, 12% from Western Europe (mostly The Netherlands), 11% from the Middle East, and 12% from Australia. Most (83%) were from university departments and medical schools (although multidisciplinary authorship where some authors were not working in academic units was common). About 26% of these articles reported clinical studies, 16% were reports of research into delivery of care, and 5% were on prescribing. Research methodology was the subject of 7%, and a further 2% dealt with providing support for research and organizations. Over the review period and beyond, the acceptance rate for papers in *Family Practice* has been in the region of 40%, and I frequently have the experience of rejecting perfectly publishable material simply because of space and the shape, balance, and content of the next issue of the journal. It is clear that changes in the research culture of primary care will need to be accompanied by greater opportunities for dissemination.

Basic Principles of Effective Dissemination

The following sections will outline some basic principles and then consider in more detail different formats for presentation.

The effective presentation and communication of any research material demands the acquisition and use of good communication skills, which, although varying with the medium—paper, oral presentation, poster, or report—share many common and important principles. Perhaps the most important of these is clarity in telling the intended audience why the study you are about to report was undertaken in the first place. The context in which the study was conceived, planned, and conducted has to be made explicit so that the audience can quickly judge whether this is likely to be a question of relevance or interest to them, and to engage their attention. Access to a critical, constructive, and trusting group of colleagues is of prime importance here, with candid comments at an early stage often preventing wasted hours and disappointment.

The traditional "IMRD" structure of scientific papers—Introduction, Methods, Results, Discussion—summarizes an enduring framework into which much of the output of primary care research can be fitted. The Introduction tells the audience why the subject was chosen for study and what the study set out to do. The Methods section describes how the study was conducted, in enough detail for someone else with similar interests to determine the validity and appropriateness of the methods used. The Results section presents the findings of the research and comments on their validity and reliability, but leaves the Discussion for comments on their significance, the way they are likely to have an impact on practice, and the next steps to be taken.

In addition to this structured approach to the arrangement of a research communication, at least two other steps are of crucial importance. The first is to research the medium being used. Be sure about the content and focus of the meeting or journal you have in mind, and in your cover letter tell the selection committee or journal editor why your contribution should be chosen. Avoid verbosity and excessive claims to originality, but remember that editors and review panels will likely know far less about the subject than you do, so tell them in clear and concise language why your presentation should be of interest to readers. Second, ensure that your data are clear and comprehensible. The best way to do this is to discuss the results beforehand with informed colleagues. A departmental run-through, where colleagues are able to comment on your presentation in good time for modification before a meeting or on your draft paper before submission, is invaluable and is just as important for department chairs as it is for junior research fellows. People who do not rehearse their talks or circulate draft papers often have anxieties that they mistakenly hope can be glossed over when the time comes. Familiarity with your own material is likely to be weakly correlated with your ability to communicate it to others, so be prepared for bafflement, and see it as a means to getting helpful suggestions for modification and clarification.

OPTIMIZING PRESENTATION

The following are basic guidelines and in themselves are no guarantee of effective and successful presentation or publication, but may help.

- *Engage your audience:* Pose a controversial question using arresting visual or written material, and communicate your own enthusiasm for the subject. Try for an interesting title, but even an uninspiring title can be transformed into an arresting presentation simply by explaining why the study is important.

- Be sure to *describe the context* of the research succinctly, so that its relevance is crystal clear. Avoid tedious reiteration of every published paper that bears on your own research—but equally, do not leave out key prior work, or you will give the impression that you do not know where you are starting from.

- *Emphasize the novelty* of your findings and try to *maintain momentum* throughout a clear presentation of your data. Enthusiasm in the presentation of both the methods, particularly when they are new, and the results, particularly when they are at odds with other data or provide answers to hitherto unresolved questions, should be communicated as forcefully as possible. Let the audience see that you are pleased with what you have done and are proud of your efforts.

- *Avoid tedious, repetitive formats,* both written and graphic, that simply lull the reader or the audience into non-attention. Recapitulate the key findings, relate them to your original research question, and finally comment on them in a way that will stimulate thought, generate interest, and, if at all possible, evoke admiration. Self-effacement is one thing, but try not to hide your light under a bushel of modesty and uncertainty.

- Finally, when presenting at meetings, *try to be available* at the end of the session for informal discussion with interested colleagues—and, for the career-minded, for discussion with senior faculty from your next target institution!

STYLE

In both oral and written work, pay attention to grammatical style. The subjunctive voice (it was considered appropriate . . . it was found to be more significant . . .) and other stylized and traditional medical modes are inelegant and frequently disliked by editors, and anyway are inappropriate for oral presentations. Phrases such as "we wondered whether there might be a connection between . . . " or "it seemed likely that . . . " are more naturalistic, appealing, and digestible than stodgy medicoscientific prose.

Edward Huth, who edited the *Annals of Internal Medicine*, has written an invaluable book on writing and publishing papers in the medical sciences (Huth, 1990). His five targets for good scientific prose are *fluency, clarity, accuracy, economy,* and *grace*. Fluency depends on paragraph length, connections, and structure, and sentence structure and length. Clarity frequently suffers from misplaced modifying words or phrases, ambiguities, and the wrong choice of verb tenses. The main ingredient of accuracy is correct use of scientific nomenclature and careful choice of words to avoid misuse. (Also be careful, of course, to avoid spelling errors, which become increasingly difficult to spot with each rereading of the manuscript. Spell-check functions on word processors can help.) Economy means tightly written prose, with excision of unneeded words and phrases and replacement of long words with shorter equivalents. Avoid excessive use of weak verbs, abstract nouns, superfluous clauses, and empty phrases and words. Grace has to do not only with the avoidance of dehumanizing words, pomposity, slang, and jargon, but probably also includes a sizeable component of unlearnable literary elegance. We should remember Samuel Johnson's comment that "most editors are failed authors . . . but again, so are most authors."

Huth's book is essential and entertaining reading for us all, containing as it does gems such as the "so-what" test, the "who-cares" test, and an invaluable list of "Twenty Steps in Planning, Writing and Publishing a Paper," which takes the researcher from the first step of deciding on the message to the delicious final state of awaiting publication.

SPECIAL CASES

Presentation and dissemination may be further optimized by bearing in mind a number of tips and wrinkles relating to specific modes of communication.

Abstracts

Fewer and fewer meetings play the traditional abstract game, it seems, and promises of Nobel-standard revelations are less acceptable than real data. In many ways this is a pity, not least because it tends to prolong the agony between doing a study and reporting it, but conference-organizing committees have their problems too. When submitting an abstract, clarify the type of presentation it is for (e.g., plenary or parallel session, poster, workshop) and tailor your submission accordingly, bearing in mind how long you will have available to speak. Slick parallel sessions of 10-minutes-for-presentation-5-for-discussion-and-on-to-the-next-paper do not suit all of us, and are particularly useless for discussions of pilot studies and work in progress. The conference organizers who will be reviewing your abstract do not have much to go on, so think hard about your title and consider making a statement about your results rather than saying what kind of study you did. Don't be gimmicky, but don't be dull. Stick exactly to the abstract guidelines and be prepared to buy your secretary flowers when you see the final, word-perfect version sitting just inside the blue box. Take the deadline seriously. Consider what you will do if you do not get an oral presentation but are offered a poster; the production of a good research poster can be more difficult than the weightiest keynote address, and merits at least a chapter in another book.

Oral Presentations

Once the abstract has been accepted there will be a period of frantic activity to verify the hastily assembled data included in it and to do the statistics properly. You are likely to have 10 minutes to tell a waiting world about your work. The main message has to be, "Don't go it alone." Unless you are very experienced, the development and delivery of a 10-minute presentation will be infinitely better if it is rehearsed, revised, and rehearsed again, with comments coming in from your coworkers and, importantly, from colleagues less familiar with the research area.

Well before you present, familiarize yourself with your chairperson and with the audiovisual system in the room in which you will be speaking. Check that slides are oriented correctly, that there is a pointer of some kind, that you know how to change the slides and lighting, and—crucial, if you are in a large room—what effect turning away from the microphone has on the sound system and on your audibility.

With regard to slides, there is rarely time to indulge in a moody photographic study of your home town or institution, but always time for a good title slide that tells the audience what the study is called, who did it, and where it was done. (It is also perfectly permissible and often highly effective to precede the title slide with some contextual comments about why the study needed to be done, either with a slide or two or with the lights on.)

Keep the slides clear and simple. How often have you heard prestigious presenters apologizing for slides? In an age of superb graphics packages, it is inexcusable and embarrassing to hear comments such as "I don't expect you can read that at the back, but don't worry about the details," or "I'm sorry that the pink doesn't show up very well," but of course we will continue to do so. Try to keep the color scheme uniform, and avoid luridness and dark colors, which project badly.

There are plenty of rules but few certainties about how much you should put on each slide. Present numerical data sparingly and crisply, and think about how much narrative you want on your slides—it might be better just to say something. Do not put on material that you do not refer to orally: Talk to the slide on the screen. The most ghastly misunderstandings can arise from a mismatch between the oral and visual message from the platform. Also, always assume that your audience is half asleep. Keep them awake, explain everything, keep moving.

Display the hypothesis or research question, aims and objectives, and methods and results, and leave time for at least one conclusion slide and preferably one for a couple of pithy comments saying where we should go from here. Try to end on an upbeat and positive note; do not trail off with a weak comment about that being just about all you've got to say. Approach reserve slides for question time with trepidation; unless you have briefed a projectionist, you may spend the whole discussion session flicking back and forth looking for the right slide.

The Research Paper

Once you have satisfied the who-cares and so-what criteria, the next step is to decide on the appropriate journal. This is not as easy as it seems, if some of the curious submissions received by editors are anything to go by. Take advice from experienced colleagues, and go over the past year or so's issues to get a clear idea of the material of interest and, in the case of less familiar journals, to avoid duplicating recent publications. Much of the detail—the structure of the paper and the abstract, its length, style of text, tables, figures, and references—will follow from reviewing the journal and from reading its instructions to authors. Even if some of these instructions seem niggling, do not ignore them, because they have usually been put there for a good reason; follow them to the letter.

The paper will go through drafts and rewrites in response to your coauthors' and others' views and comments, but during this painful process keep in mind some factors that might enhance the chances of acceptance. Follow the basic principles described earlier and pay attention to Huth's (1990) criteria for good prose style. Make the title count—it should never be neutral, but do not overdo it—and ensure that the introduction makes the rationale for doing your study and its principal aims crystal clear. Do not skimp on the methods section (there should be enough there to enable someone else to repeat your work), and highlight key results: Avoid diluting them in a lot of less enthralling data. Do not reiterate text in tables and vice versa: Use figures if they are easier to understand than tables, but keep both uncluttered and focused. Do not go on forever in the discussion; be candid about possible methodological limitations of your work and its relationship to other published evidence. Keep the discussion on track and end with some ideas about next steps and developments.

Just as with an oral presentation, the presentation of your paper matters. Word processors and printers are capable of producing material that is attractive, well laid out, correctly spelled, and easy to read. Avoid bizarre fonts. Make sure there is a front sheet with title, authors, institution, and correspondence address. Ensure that line spacing is correct, margins adequate, pages numbered, figures and tables correctly captioned, and references correctly arranged, and send the right number of copies.

In the cover letter, avoid both obsequiousness and grandiosity, but say why the paper is worth publishing and why the particular journal has been selected. Do get the editor's name, initials, institute, and postal address correct (I have a personal aversion to papers submitted to an anagram of my name at a novel medical school address).

Conclusion

For writing, presenting, and publishing, and for the doing of the research itself, isolation is the deadliest enemy. The physical isolation of the lone practice-based researcher is the most extreme example but, for a host of reasons, we all put fences up and develop idiosyncratic sensitivities. Membership in a trusting, friendly, bright, and skeptical group of researchers may be the best defense against isolation. Nobody started out in research with a long curriculum vitae, and we have all suffered at the hands of reviewers, editors, and conference subversives. Good and effective dissemination depends on good people doing good work and talking to each other about it.

References

Haynes, R. B. (1990). Loose connections between peer-reviewed clinical journals and clinical practice. *Annals of Internal Medicine, 113*(9), 724-728.

Huth, E. J. (1990). *How to write and publish papers in the medical sciences* (2nd ed.). Baltimore, MD: Williams & Wilkins.

Jones, R. (1990). International family practice research. *Family Practice, 7,* 75-76.

Jones, R. (1991). European General Practice Research Workshop. *Family Practice, 8,* 111.

Jones, R., Wilmot, J., & Fry, J. (1991). The General Practice Research Club. *British Journal of General Practice, 41,* 380-381.

McWhinney, I. R. (1991). Primary care research in the next twenty years. In P. G. Norton, M. Stewart, F. Tudiver, M. J. Bass, & E. V. Dunn (Eds.), *Primary care research: Traditional and innovative approaches* (pp. 1-12). Newbury Park, CA: Sage.

Peckham, M. (1991). *Research for health.* London: HMSO.

5 Disseminating Qualitative Research

JANICE M. MORSE

"I can't hear you while I'm listening!"

The above paradox was the title of a phenomenological study by Baron (1985), who found himself using these words while listening intently through a stethoscope. His qualitative article describes the preoccupation of physicians with the technical/diagnostic aspects of care at the expense of the patient's reports and consideration of the patient as a person.

Qualitative research is powerful. When communicated clearly, the results of a qualitative study reach us, and, for instance, may make us uncomfortable, for we may be all guilty of listening too intently to hear. Whereas quantitative results merge responses so that if only 5% of the sample were "satisfied" with the service, then at least it is comforting to know that the needs of 5% were being satisfied. Qualitative research results may be so direct, so on target, that those who have participated may have "nowhere to hide" (Miles, personal communication, October 1992).

In this chapter the techniques of disseminating qualitative research findings effectively will be discussed. Some of the difficulties in getting qualitative ideas into writing; certain conventions and nuances that writers should be aware of; issues, such as editing quotes, maintaining anonymity, and in presenting negative findings; and issues specific to different modes of dissemination will be discussed.

Writing Up Qualitative Research

The nature of qualitative research and the fact that its data are collected, stored, and retrieved as descriptive text, lulls the researcher into a false expectation that, after months of recording, reporting will be easy. In this section, some of the potential difficulties will be explored and techniques to facilitate the writing process and communicate qualitative findings clearly and effectively will be outlined.

GETTING STARTED

Some time ago, I received an invitation to serve as a consultant for a postdoctoral program. "Our qualitative researchers," I was told, "are having trouble writing up their data." The qualitative researcher does not "write up" data. Rather, qualitative researchers write up the *analysis* that should be at some level of interpretation and abstraction beyond the interview text. Reports should not simply consist of quotations linked together with minimal textual commentary. Thus, perhaps the greatest cause of writer's block is prematurely attempting to write before completing the analysis; that is, before developing and finalizing the emerging theory and connecting it with the work of others. Until the analysis is complete, how will the researcher know what to write?

One helpful approach is, before beginning to write, to present or explain the theory to colleagues. Somehow, putting one's thoughts into words eases the process of putting the words onto paper. Furthermore, questions that arise from the discussion may assist the researcher to see any gaps or conceptually thin areas where the reasoning is not quite clear. In addition, the process of explaining the results and responding to questions helps to clarify the theory for the researcher. And, assuming that "two (plus) heads are better than one," the theoretical knowledge of colleagues may provide new conceptual linkages that increase the theoretical generalizability of the study, thereby making it stronger and more significant than realized. Colleagues may be experts in qualitative methods or know nothing of its methods and assumptions; they may be familiar or unfamiliar with the topic; they may be clinical experts in the area or know little about it—for the most fruitful discussion, a mixed seminar is best.

EDITING QUOTES

In order to maintain the integrity of the data during the analysis phase, when transcribing conversations with participants it is important that all of the interview material be transcribed verbatim. To enable the researcher to continue to "hear" the interview, indicate pauses and include all expressions in the text. Placing unedited transcription directly into the document adds nothing to the reader's appreciation of the results: in fact, the opposite occurs. Rather than illustrating a particular point and making your intended message clearer, an unedited quote filled with irrelevant material distracts the reader, obscures the message, and may even be so difficult to read that the reader will skip it altogether.

The question is, how to cull the quotations and still maintain the integrity of the data? Standard punctuation conventions usually are sufficient to indicate to readers that editing has taken place (Field & Morse, 1985). For example, if only part of a quotation is needed, replace the irrelevant part with three ellipsis points (. . .) to indicate text deleted from within a sentence, or four ellipsis points to indicate a deletion between two sentences. A pause may be indicated by a long dash (—) and a thoughtful, lengthy pause may be shown in square bracket as: [long pause]. Any emotional reactions that are necessary to include may be inserted inside square brackets, as: [laughs] or [crying]. Square brackets may also be used to indicate who is being referred to when the person's name is removed, such as: "J [brother]." If participants make grammatical errors when speaking, these should remain but be acknowledged with a "[sic]." Accents are more difficult to transcribe and should be transcribed with care to avoid insulting the ethnic group whose dialect is being phonetically written. Furthermore, if only one of the participants in the setting has an accent, adding this characteristic to the quotation may identify the speaker to all readers familiar with the setting, thus violating the researcher's agreement to conceal participants' identities. This issue is explored in more detail below.

BUILDING YOUR CASE

There are two basic styles of presenting qualitative work. The first is to present a synopsis or overview of the resulting theory—to serve as a guide for the reader—and then follow this with the supporting data. The second style is to present the results as the theory was developed, so that the reader shares the insights and the conclusions, bit by bit, step by step. In both cases, by the time the readers have reached the end of the results section, they will share the researcher's insights and conclusions.

The conclusions should be clear, with alternative explanations and hypotheses systematically excluded, and with in-depth descriptions that vividly portray each point. Judiciously added examples—informants' quotes, exemplars, and case histories—provide richness. Subheadings should be used to keep the reader on track and to highlight each point.

USING QUOTES

The effective use of participants' quotes is important, but should only be used if a participant has made a point in a manner better than could be expressed by the researcher. Except in the case of presenting unwelcome results (as discussed below), each point should be clearly described before the quote is used, so that the quote simply serves as an illustration. The full range of diversity, or the characteristics and the synthesis of all the material pertaining to that section, should be included in the text. Remember that the quote supplements the text and provides human insight and dimension to the analysis. As discussed, quotes may be edited and extraneous material removed.

One of the most common mistakes made by new researchers is that they consider almost all their data to be significant and all their quotes vital. A suggestion that any of the quotes are redundant or insufficiently important and should be removed is met with a storm of protest. Remember: It is easier to be tough on yourself than to have an article rejected.

DIAGRAMMING, MODELING, AND THE
USE OF TABLES

The presentation of some qualitative methods is particularly enhanced by the use of diagramming, modeling, or the effective use of tables to provide overviews or schemes of the study. These serve to keep the reader on track and often attract the attention of the casual reader flipping through a journal. They may even assist in the process of writing up the research, by preventing derailments or diversions to less significant material while the article is being outlined.

Grounded theory research is particularly suited to diagramming, as the end product is substantive or formal theory (see, e.g., Chenitz & Swanson, 1986). The stages, phases, and strategies of each part may be listed in a summary or the model may be diagrammed with the direction and processes of the BSP (Basic Social Process) or the BSPP (Basic Social Psychological Process) explicated with arrows (see, e.g., Morse & Johnson, 1991). Ethnography is also often easily diagrammed with the characteristics of each category listed in a table (see, e.g., the taxonomies of ethnoscience in Spradley and McCurdy, 1972).

SOME CONVENTIONS OF QUALITATIVE WRITING

In all writing, start by identifying the audience. This will ensure that not only the content, but also the language and style, are targeted to the reader (see the section on "Identifying the Audience").

When presenting qualitative reports, be sensitive to the various voices in the text and be careful to separate the informant's perspective (the emic voice) from the researcher's view (the etic voice) and the analytic comment. If these distinctions are not explicit, the presentation can be confusing for the reader and appear as poor science. One strategy is to separate the perspectives under different subheadings so that there is no doubt as to who or what is being presented.

Issues of mixing perspectives can to some extent affect the style of writing. Some authors prefer to write in the first person in order to make the ethnographic report more personal, and others elect to present the data in the third person or even to omit any reference to the researcher. The style that is used is personal choice, but, before beginning it is wise to check the author's guidelines of the selected journal, in case the editor has set a style for the publication.

Qualitative researchers use quotation marks frequently in their writing to draw the reader's attention to a common word that is being used uncommonly. The quotation marks may denote that the word is being used in a special way by participants or may denote a particular meaning. Minnich (1990, p. xvi) refers to the latter case as "scare quotes" to indicate that the words are being used deliberately, "self-consciously," where specific language is used for the reader to hear "as it vibrates between levels and across situations and realms of meaning." This particular use of quotations is problematic for copy editors who are unfamiliar with qualitative work, and may not recognize their significance.

MAINTAINING PARTICIPANT ANONYMITY

One important task when writing up qualitative research is to maintain the anonymity and all other agreements made at the time the research was negotiated. This includes not revealing the identity of the participants or of the institution and frequently even the location or city in which the research was conducted. It is wise to have your report read carefully by a colleague to confirm that anonymity has been maintained.

Note that even if you ensure anonymity, if you intend to quote participants' words, complete confidentiality cannot be ensured. Consent forms should make this risk clear. Suggested wording might be:

> Our conversation will be tape-recorded and transcribed. Your name will not be on the transcription, associated with the study, or on any publication resulting from this research; however, some of your words may be included in these reports.

What must be recognized is that even though names are removed from all quotations, the presence of "tags" and other identifiers may enable people involved in the research—including other participants—to link identifiers and thus reconstruct informants' identities. The more tags or links left by the investigator, the easier this process may be and the greater the risk of exposure for the participants when the report is disseminated. Therefore, it is recommended that as few identifiers as possible be placed in the report. Strategies that may be used include:

1. Report only aggregate demographic information, such as ages in ranges. Especially if the number of participants is less than 10, do not prepare a table that lists age, marital status, sex, ethnicity, and so forth person by person. Determining who participated in the study and who did not is then only a matter of elimination for those familiar with the research setting.
2. Do not place an identifier at the end of each quote, even if it is a pseudonym. Often a quote may be linked to a participant by a single comment, and such a clue would then enable someone to link and pool all quotations published from that person's interviews.
3. If it is important to place some identifiers at the end of each quotation, such as age and sex of the speaker, then it is permissible to systematically change all ages by a few years, just as it is permissible to provide pseudonyms or to change the names of cities to protect the participants. But be sure to alert the reader in a footnote to the fact that these details have been changed in the report.

Remember, in qualitative research the sample probably was selected to participate in the study not because of particular demographic characteristics such as age or sex, but rather because of some other life experience. (For example, a researcher studying the coping strategies of spinal cord injury patients may select subjects on the basis of whether or not they have remained hopeful and have coped well on discharge.) Glaser (1978) argues that demographic characteristics should not be considered significant until they emerge as such and have earned their way into the emerging model. The compulsion to report these factors may have been acquired from our quantitative colleagues and may jeopardize the anonymity of our sample, while contributing little toward the replicability of the study.

REPORTING NEGATIVE FINDINGS

One of the most difficult tasks in writing up qualitative results is to maintain validity: to remain, as Bergum (1989/1991) describes it, "true to their words" (p. 54) and to include aspects that are negative, uncomplimentary, or critical in the final report. A problem may arise when these results have to be reported back to the agency or institution where the study was conducted, and may not be received graciously by (or may even offend) those who had permitted the access. On the one hand it is both immoral and against research ethics not to report problems the study revealed; on the other hand, by reporting them, there is a risk of alienating your "host."

The first task is to prevent the fear of offending from looming so large as to prevent anything from being written at all. Write the first draft as well as possible, with descriptive fairness that does justice to the research. Then explain your dilemma to a colleague whose judgment may be trusted, and ask that person to read the draft, flagging anything that may be offensive or problematic. It is possible that you are simply being overly sensitive to the whole matter, and few, if any, changes will be required. If changes are necessary it will probably be a simple matter to write the critical portions more softly, or with more justification, so that the conclusions are evident. Alternatively, limit the negative comments to the quotations, so that they are all attributed to the participants. If worse comes to worst, consult with a lawyer before releasing the findings; however, there is no guarantee that this will prevent problems, such as subpoena of data to "confirm the findings" as Barinaga's (1992) report on DiFranza et al.'s research on "Old Joe Camel" recently revealed.

Another strategy may be to "test the waters" by presenting the findings to a trusted contact in the host organization. It is possible that the organization may be aware of the problem but not the underlying cause and be grateful for the information. Alternatively, the contact person may be able to diffuse the findings at the board meeting when the results are to be presented, so that the raw truth does not appear so shocking.

When presenting, the use of the royal "we" (i.e., including oneself as a fellow human stuck in the same dilemma) may soften the blow and help develop a more constructive attitude toward the results. And, if there is absolutely no way around the problem, take a colleague with you when presenting—someone to pick up the pieces, buy you a drink, and drive you home.

Effective Oral Presentations

GIVING TALKS

Superficially, talking about qualitative findings should be easier than talking about quantitative ones, as qualitative findings are not usually hampered with tables, graphs, charts, and figures. Theoretically, qualitative research lends itself naturally to "story-telling," to verbal presentation.

Unfortunately, this is not always the case, because there is rarely enough time in a 15-minute presentation to present a comprehensive, complete study. Thus the researcher is forced artificially to focus and present one narrow portion of it. Invariably, a member of the audience will ask, "What about . . .," and the researcher will predictably respond, "Well, I do have that included in my model, but there wasn't enough time to discuss it." Qualitative data cannot be presented as neatly and efficiently as in quantitative tables and figures; rather, the context must be described, the participants' experiences explained, quotes read, and the emerging theory explicated.

Slides or overheads can do much to facilitate this process and help the listener grasp the main points. If participants' quotes are shown on slides, the listener can read the words with the presenter and thus add more meaning to the presentation. Try to use stories and exemplars to illustrate powerful points. They can make the participants come alive, and most importantly, longer stories related in qualitative presentations may be profoundly moving.

PREPARING POSTERS

Practical hints for the preparation of research posters are described in detail elsewhere (Bushy, 1991; Kirkpatrick & Martin, 1991; Lippman & Ponton, 1989). Briefly, view your poster as would a conference participant—that is, check how it reads from a distance of 4 feet and in a period of 3 or 4 minutes. The poster should be laid out sequentially so that it makes sense to someone walking by and draw in those interested in the topic. Colors should be attractive and the type large enough to be easily read (18-point bold font is ideal).

Qualitative results take up more space than a quantitative summary. Thus, when preparing a poster, put the emphasis on the findings. Depending on the qualitative methods used, emphasize the categories developed and the relationships between them. Because the context is significant it should also be described.

Diagram the models used. Photographs really catch attention: A picture says a thousand words. If the qualitative study does not lend itself to being presented on tables or figures, a brief but significant informant's quotation may be used to illustrate a category and to provide a direct, clear message.

VIDEOS

As a means of presenting qualitative research, videos may be a most powerful technique because they enable the viewer to see and understand the setting and the experience. To summarize research results as a video documentary complete with commentary, however, is extraordinarily expensive and time consuming.

An alternative may be to use a video just to illustrate an oral presentation, while you provide the commentary, the interpretation, or analysis—over the audio portion, or turn the sound off altogether. This technique provides the presenter with more versatility, as portions of the video may be selected and substituted as the focus of the presentation changes.

Timing of the video segments and the presentation is important, so practice to ensure that the presentation will fill the allocated time. Once your presentation has begun, the time is "fixed" and cannot be hurried or extended—only terminated if there is insufficient time to complete the presentation.

Getting Published

BOOKS AND MONOGRAPHS

Qualitative research is best disseminated as book-length manuscripts, as this gives enough space to really tell the reader what was found. Books do have some disadvantages: Often they do not have the rigorous review that an article undergoes and therefore are not as highly regarded in some universities as refereed articles.

Further, they are not accessed as easily as articles through such bibliographic retrieval services as Medline where one can locate an article by author, title, or topic and obtain a copy of the abstract on-line.

The advantages, however, are tremendous; the main advantage is that once a contract is obtained, the publication of the book is more or less ensured. Also, a year or two after publication, royalties may even be awarded.

Obtaining a Contract

Unlike the rules for journal articles, it is permissible and prudent to approach several publishers simultaneously to determine their preliminary interest in publishing the manuscript. Invariably, a proposal will be requested. The editor will provide you with specific instructions for preparing the proposal. Basically, a proposal should consist of the title and a few paragraphs about the book; a table of contents; a few paragraphs about you as an author stating your writing experience, why the book is unique, what its competing volumes are, and why you are qualified to write it; and some completed sample chapters. The publisher may send copies of your proposal to experts nationwide for review and comment.

Publishing Articles

To split or not to split: Frequently, the first decision to be made when preparing an article for publication is to delineate its content; that is to "split" a report or dissertation into publishable, manageable units. The goal is to maintain significant content and focus in each article, without "over-diluting" by turning the report into too many articles so that none has adequate theory or substance to stand alone. There is often pressure on junior faculty to err on the side of more publications, for in the "publish or perish" context, the number of articles, rather than their substance, is valued for achieving tenure and promotion. Yet, journal editors are suspicious of articles that refer to several others that appear to be similar, being concerned about copyright violation and preferring to publish really original work. If the author goes on to write several articles around the first one published, editors realize that subsequent articles must cite or otherwise acknowledge the first.

Presenting papers at conferences prior to submitting them for publications will assist in the identification of areas of interest to your colleagues, and from the questions and responses of the audience will provide some "feel" for whether the areas will be able to stand alone. Using this feedback, it is wise to deliberately plan the content of each paper, rather than to let it simply "emerge." The order in which the articles are submitted for publication is important; essential papers may then be referred to as "in press."

Identifying the Audience

The journal readership is most important to consider before submitting an article, for it will determine the focus and the style of the writing. Does the audience consist of researchers or clinicians? If they are researchers, are they experienced investigators who will not require much in-depth explanation of the methods, or are they new to research and require a clear and detailed explanation? If they are clinicians, do they consist primarily of physicians, nurses, other health professionals, or a mixture of these disciplines? Are the implications for practice clearly written, along with any caveats or concerns?

Choosing the Journal

Some journal editors have implemented regulations that weaken the reporting of qualitative research. Most common is an insistence on restricting the length of submissions to 15 pages (often less). This results in difficulties for qualitative submissions, for rarely can all the requirements for the richness of description be developed in a short article. Other editors may insist that a certain outline be strictly adhered to, and this outline might not be conducive to the presentation of qualitative reporting. For example, the requirement that a literature review must be presented before the results may not be ideal for a study using grounded theory, when linkage to the literature is inherent within the presentation of results. van Manen (1984) notes that presentation of a research question and description of the method are not necessary for phenomenology—such sections make for an unnecessary distraction from the poetics of the writing.

Another case may be made for describing the method only when it deviates from a standard description that is more clearly presented in a methodology text. For instance, reading summary after similar summary of grounded theory in article after article is really unnecessary, when the reader could as easily be referred to Strauss (1987) or Strauss and Corbin (1990). Space in journals is too expensive for such reiterations, and the same standards of explication are not required of quantitative researchers. As May (1991) notes, quantitative researchers may briefly describe their method and provide a citation, and these same standards should be acceptable for qualitative researchers.

When to Submit?

When the article is completed, put it away and read it again after a day or two. Read it out loud. Does it say what was intended? Or is another draft necessary? Check for consistency—does the title match the purpose and fit what the article is about? Check for balance—is the bulk of the article about the topic? Check the format with the author's guidelines for the journal. And finally, run a spell-check before the final printing.

A smart researcher never sends an article to a publisher without both a peer review (for content) and an editor's check (for style and format) (see Morse, 1993). Fresher or sharper eyes may spot areas of weakness, omissions, and other problems in the manuscript that were hidden from you and would be embarrassing if you sent them out uncorrected.

The Nitty-Gritty of Format

Meeting format requirements is really a technical task, but a correct format is important. If it is neglected or unsatisfactory, the article will be sent back to you for corrections and may not make it to press.

One of the most common and careless errors is that authors do not send all their pages to the editor, or leave off a figure—most often lost during copying. Occasionally the editor notices and can fax the missing page; more often a reviewer notes it, and the whole process is delayed while the reviewer notifies the editor, who notifies the author, who mails the missing item to the editor, who mails it on to the reviewers, who then continue with the review.

A second problem is the use of a poor quality printer to produce the final version. Dot matrix type does not copy well, especially if the ribbon is not new. Use a laser printer even if one is not easily accessible. Reviewers must be able to read what they are evaluating. Also remember that most journals require that documents be double-spaced to give the editor room to work, whether to add, delete, or alter the text. Everything must be double-spaced, including quotes and references.

Checking the reference list for completeness is vital. Most journals restrict the reference list to those sources cited, and, for space reasons, some even restrict the number of citations. It is most important that the format of the references match that requested by the journal, for the typesetters will enter what they see. If the format differs from that of the journal, the editor may conclude that the article must have been rejected by another journal and that the author did not even bother to disguise this fact by changing the style. The editor will then be in a mind-set to "find error" when reading the manuscript and, perhaps unfairly, assume that there must be some fatal flaw with it.

Finally, when submitting (and only to one journal at a time, please), ensure that the requested number of copies are submitted. (Editors resent having to do photocopying, as they feel they have more to do with their time and the department's funding.) Slide your submission into the mail slot with a wish, watch for an acknowledgment of its receipt, and inquire about its status if too many months go by.

DEALING WITH EDITORS AND REVIEWERS

"I like what you say, but hate the way you write."

Be aware that most editors have pet peeves and their own preferred styles. Sometimes they are "up front" with these quirks and will list them in their style sheets; other times authors may discover them serendipitously by attending a workshop or meeting others who have previously published in that journal. Not uncommonly, authors may discover these preferences the hard way, when their edited manuscripts are returned.

What are these fads? They may be minor things such as ensuring that a title does not include a colon and a subtitle, or refusing to accept the passive voice. Sometimes these revisions may result in major changes or in rejection of the article. Some editors will not consider qualitative studies, just as *Qualitative Health Research* does not publish quantitative research. When selecting a journal, review previous issues to see how the articles are directed, how they are presented, and if qualitative research has been published in that particular venue.

Responding to Reviewers

One of the more delicate tasks of the editor is to serve as a mediator between the reviewers and the author, to evaluate the reviewers' remarks, and to make a decision on whether to accept, reject, or to request revisions on an article. The editor may summarize the comments and give very clear directive to the author, or may simply forward all the comments. In the latter case, some of the reviewers' remarks/criticisms may be contradictory—one reviewer may write complimentary remarks about a particular passage, and a second may pull it to shreds and request it to be revised. Should you be caught between two conflicting positions, the onus is on you to respond either by revising the article, or by responding to the editor in a cover letter ("I concur with Reviewer A and have not altered the third paragraph; Reviewer B is apparently not familiar with methods for selecting qualitative samples").

Remember, the author is responsible for the content of the article and part of this responsibility is to write clearly. It is important, therefore, that if some passage is unclear, to take negative criticisms very seriously and try to understand why a certain point was unclear or misinterpreted.

MANAGING PROOFS

When an article is returned as page proofs, be sure to check pages carefully. Some editors will publish a manuscript as is, simply checking to ensure that the reference list is correct, whereas others may rewrite the article. The latter approach is particularly troublesome for authors, as the meaning intended by the author may be subtly changed and the text is painstakingly difficult to check with the original.

Although seemingly months may have passed since the article was submitted, publishers may require the return of the corrected proofs within 48 hours. This is simply the nature of publishing, and the deadline must be kept. Extension should only be requested in extraordinary circumstances.

Summary

Writing qualitative research does require a different approach from writing quantitative research, and adhering to a few simple principles will help the process go more smoothly. First, complete the analysis before beginning to write. Be clear about what is to be written, and select and edit all the quotes to be included before beginning. Identify the audience and the journal. And finally, when writing, be true to the principles of qualitative inquiry: Write with richness, with realism, and with rigor.

References

Barinaga, M. (1992) Who controls a researcher's files? *Science, 256,* 1620-1621.

Baron, R. J. (1985). An introduction to medical phenomenology: I can't hear you while I'm listening. *Annals of Internal Medicine, 103,* 606-611.

Bergum, V. (1989/1991). Being a phenomenological researcher. In J. M. Morse (Ed.), *Qualitative nursing research: A contemporary dialogue* (pp. 55-71). Newbury Park, CA: Sage.

Bushy, A. (1991). A rating scale to evaluate research poster. *Nurse Educator, 1691,* 11-15.

Chenitz, C., & Swanson, J. (1986). *From practice to grounded theory.* Menlo Park, CA: Addison-Wesley.

Field, P. A., & Morse, J. M. (1985). *Nursing research: The application of qualitative approaches.* London: Croom Helm.

Glaser, B. G. (1978). *Theoretical sensitivity.* Mill Valley, CA: Sociology Press.

Kirkpatrick, H., & Martin, M. L. (1991). Communicating nursing research through poster presentation. *Western Journal of Nursing Research, 13*(1), 145-148.

Lippman, D. T., & Ponton, K. S. (1989). Designing a research poster with impact. *Western Journal of Nursing Research, 11*(4), 477-485.

May, K. A. (1991). Dialogue: The granting game. In J. M. Morse (Ed.), *Qualitative nursing research: A contemporary dialogue* (rev. ed.) (pp. 188-201). Newbury Park, CA: Sage.

Minnich, E. K. (1990). *Transforming knowledge.* Philadelphia: Temple University Press.

Morse, J. M. (1993). The perfect manuscript. *Qualitative Health Research, 3,* 3-5.

Morse, J. M., & Johnson, J. (1991). *The illness experience: Dimensions of suffering.* Newbury Park, CA: Sage.

Spradley, J. P., & McCurdy, D. W. (1972). *The cultural experience.* Kingsport, TN: Kingsport Press.

Strauss, A. (1987). *Qualitative analysis for social scientists.* Cambridge: Cambridge University Press.

Strauss, A., & Corbin, J. (1990). *Basics of qualitative research.* Newbury Park, CA: Sage.

van Manen, M. (1984). Practicing phenomenological writing. *Phenomenology and Pedagogy, 1,* 3669.

6 The Media and the
Dissemination of Research

PETER DESBARATS

As I began to think about this chapter, I recalled a conversation about 8 years ago with one of my graduate journalism students who had come to us with an undergraduate degree in science. He was trying to provide me with an explanation of the difference between journalistic and scientific mentalities.

As a science student, he explained, he had learned that scientific research requires a narrow and consistent focus of attention on a relatively small aspect of reality. About halfway through his studies, however, he started to write stories about science for campus newspapers. This required him to take a broader perspective, to range widely among various scientific interests, and to communicate rapidly and clearly. The articles that he wrote had to be interesting, even entertaining; and because of the pressure of writing to inflexible deadlines, he often had time to gain only a relatively superficial knowledge of his subjects.

Despite these drawbacks, perhaps even because of them, he found that he was attracted to journalism. Science began to appear limiting and narrow compared with the wide-ranging and comparatively undisciplined work of the journalist. This was the way he defined the difference between the two mentalities. The last I heard of him, he was working in the information service of a large university, producing articles about scientific research.

This chapter will survey some of the most recent expert observations about the communication of science. My approach will be to examine the wider field of scientific and medical news coverage in general, and then to attempt to apply some of my observations and conclusions to the problem of disseminating primary care research through the news media. Because I still consider myself to be primarily a journalist, the chapter will be catholic in its approach, anecdotal, and, I hope, at least interesting (if not irresistibly entertaining).

In my search for articles, I was assisted by the Journalism Periodical Index of the Graduate School of Journalism at The University of Western Ontario. This is a unique database that contains more than 18,000 references to articles about news media in popular and academic periodicals, primarily in North America. A search for items related to science, medical, or health journalism produced more than 100 articles published since 1980; from these, I selected 40 that seemed relevant. Perhaps significantly, none of the articles was devoted specifically to the relationship between primary care research and the news media, although many of them related to the work of primary care physicians.

The Two Solitudes of Journalism and Science

My starting point, as I indicated at the outset, is the inherent difference between journalists and scientists. We see an indication of this every year at the Graduate School when we select 40 students for our Master's program from about 250 qualified applicants. Very few of these ever have science degrees; the vast majority have undergraduate degrees in the humanities or social sciences, particularly—not surprisingly—in English Literature. In fact, having a science degree is an advantage in applying to our program, because we seek a diversity of backgrounds among our students and we know that there is always a shortage of journalists who can understand and communicate scientific knowledge. (We were surprised and delighted last year when a biochemist on leave from University Hospital in London, Ontario, applied to our program. Dr. Candace Gibson was accepted, of course, and she is one of the reasons why we have moved ahead quickly to create an elective course in medical journalism, on which I will provide more detail later.)

Many researchers, particularly in the United States, have tried to observe and analyze the differences between scientists and journalists. Part of the problem of communication between these two worlds lies in mutual ignorance. Journalists usually know as little about science as scientists understand about the processes of mass communication.

A survey in the late 1980s of 834 editors of U.S. daily newspapers revealed an embarrassing degree of ignorance about basic scientific information (Zimmerman, 1988). In this survey, undertaken by a biology professor at Ohio's Oberlin College, only half the editors disagreed strongly with the statement "dinosaurs and humans lived contemporaneously." One third of the respondents did not disagree strongly when presented with a statement that said, "the earth is approximately 6,000-20,000 years old," only 41% with "Adam and Eve were actual people," only 57% with "every word in the Bible is true," and only 48% with "most scientists are atheists." Only 42% agreed strongly with the correct statement: "The earth is approximately four billion to five billion years old."

The other side of this coin is the ignorance of scientists about news media and their inherent bias against the work of journalists. Two American journalism professors, in an article entitled "Scientific Barriers to the Popularization of Science in the Mass Media" (Dunwoody & Ryan, 1985) observed that "the training of scientists in the United States is highly structured, but most academic programs offer little or no assistance in helping neophyte scientists learn to communicate with nonscientists, including journalists" (p. 27). The authors went on to comment that "a lack of such training may be perceived as a significant barrier to these scientists' later ability and/or inclination to so communicate" (p. 27).

They also noted that, although lip service is given to the need for better public understanding of science, "there is little evidence that those scientists who do engage in such activities are rewarded within science" (Dunwoody & Ryan, 1985, p. 27). In fact, doctors who do make efforts to communicate with the public through news media may be judged negatively by their peers. The study just cited refers to an unpublished paper (Dunwoody, 1974) that describes the case of a medical researcher who agreed to talk to a local newspaper reporter about his research on inner-ear disorders. Two years later, when the researcher applied for membership in a prestigious scientific society, he was told that the use of his name in the featured newspaper article constituted a breach of the society's ethics.

The same professors, in an article in *Journalism Quarterly*, the most important academic publication for U.S. journalism educators, stated that "journalists and scientists . . . have different goals and concerns, and they tend to speak in different languages." The scientists "typically couch findings in languages that speak primarily to other scientists," but journalists "must translate scientific language into ordinary English" (Dunwoody & Ryan, 1983, p. 647). According to other researchers, this produces quite different writing styles. Bostian and Byrne (1984) stated that "journalists operate under the assumption that an active, verbal style is the best choice to make scientific material comprehensible" (pp. 676-677), but the writing of scientists "is often packed with passive and nominal constructions" (p. 677). Other researchers have noted that the "active" style of writing is not only more interesting for readers but produces greater comprehension.

In light of these differences, it isn't surprising that scientists and doctors tend to be critical of news reporting in their fields. Moore and Singletary (1985) stated that physicians were particularly critical of "sensationalism, inaccuracy, incompleteness of reports and the ignorance and lack of judgement on the part of the reporter" (p. 817) in their reactions to news stories. Earlier studies mentioned in Moore and Singletary's paper indicated that 40% to 60% of news stories about science were judged to be inaccurate by the scientists who had been the sources of information for these stories, although sometimes the inaccuracies were minor.

These studies indicate that the worlds of journalism and science, including medicine, represent the classic "two solitudes" in many respects. Of greater concern, at least to journalists, is the fact that the doctors' negative opinion of the news media is apparently shared by many members of the general public. Falk (1991) notes that a Canadian survey carried out in 1973 revealed that 43% of the respondents considered that the media were doing a poor job of covering science, and a study released by the University of Calgary in 1989, showed that 40% of Canadians still feel that way.

Disseminating Scientific and Medical
Findings Through the News Media

Although scientists, doctors, and the general public may be critical of media performance, no one denies its importance. Although researchers have long debated the relative role of news media and other information sources in modern society, we know from experience that much of our information is derived from the media and that news media are a major influence in shaping both personal behavior and political decisions. This is particularly true in the closely related fields of science, medicine, and health. Hinkle and Elliott (1989) stated flatly that "newspaper reports provide the public with most of its science news" (p. 353), and reported that in 1986 there were 66 daily newspapers in the United States with weekly science sections compared with only 19 in 1984—a phenomenal rate of increase. Researchers also discovered that the level of interest in science news was particularly strong among Americans in the 18-to-29 age group, the very group that newspapers have been losing as readers for several decades.

In our own era, television has replaced newspapers as the dominant medium of information. [A recent study by Johnson & Meishcke (1992), evaluating the use of news media by women for information about cancer, indicated that newspapers were the least preferred source of information, ranking behind magazines and television.] For several decades, survey after survey has shown that most people rely on television for most of their news and that television is regarded as the most credible news medium. Outside of its news programs, television also produces special programs related to science and medicine, particularly on the public television services of North America.

Within its limitations, television network news has been given a fairly high accuracy rating by American researchers. A 1982 survey of sources of science news stories on the three major U.S. television networks (Moore & Singletary, 1985) showed that only 14% of the sources judged them to be "somewhat inaccurate," and 48.5% stated that stories for which they were the primary source of information were "completely accurate." The most common complaint was that the air time given the story was not adequate.

One of the problems with television news is that it is even more restricted than newspapers when it comes to providing time or space for information about science and medicine and is even more subject to competitive pressures that encourage sensational treatment of information. A comprehensive analysis of American network television news, entertainment, and commercials (Turow & Coe, 1985) revealed "a huge gap between actual changes in the structure of medical care and TV's portrayal of that structure" (p. 37). This survey analyzed network programming in 1983, but I doubt that the conclusions of a similar study today would be substantially different. It showed that medical care was portrayed on television as "overwhelmingly appropriate, nonpolitical, and an unlimited resource" (Turow & Coe, 1985, p. 47). It presented illness as "acute and amenable to biomedical treatment" (p. 48). "Illness episodes emphasized the short-term and the straightforward" (p. 48), the study stated. "Even when coping was discussed, the patient's long-range plans or reintegration into society was rarely considered" (p. 48).

The study found that "all the program formats overwhelmingly failed to confront the government and corporate activities that have been changing the contemporary medical system and the public's relationship to it" (Turow & Coe, 1985, p. 49). It was suggested that this failure might relate to "the relationship that television networks and production firms have had with mainstream elements of the medical system . . . the relationship has been symbiotic, benefiting all parties" (p. 49). In an observation that is perhaps even more pertinent today than in 1985, the study suggests that critical institutional changes in American health care "will be reflected on network TV only after they have become entrenched politically" (p. 50).

Another source of information about medicine and health, sometimes overlooked, is supermarket tabloids. These are certainly not negligible, nor are they as inaccurate as many nonreaders of these tabloids might assume. A comparison by Hinkle and Elliott (1989) of space devoted to science stories in 1987 by three supermarket tabloids (*Weekly World News*, the *Star*, and the *National Enquirer*) and three mainstream newspapers (*USA Today*, *Philadelphia Inquirer*, and the *New York Times*) showed that the *Times* gave the most coverage to science stories, but that it was closely followed by the *Star* and the *National Enquirer*. Furthermore, the *Enquirer* devoted more than 80% of its science coverage to medical stories, compared to only 38.5% of the science stories in the *New York Times*.

A comparison of the accuracy of the medical stories in the *National Enquirer* and the mainstream press by one of our graduate students revealed few differences (Hallihan, 1988). This is not as surprising as it might seem, according to the editor of the *Enquirer* in a recent lecture to the Graduate School at the University of Western Ontario (Calder, 1993). He explained that the *Enquirer* refers all medical stories for approval to leading health organizations in the United States, and also carefully drew a distinction between his paper's medical stories and those appearing in even racier tabloids specializing in what he termed "fantasy journalism." With a weekly circulation of more than 4 million copies, the *Enquirer* may be North America's most important newspaper source of information about medicine and health.

Judging from the articles I surveyed, criticism of science and medical reporting tends to veer back and forth between two apparently opposite poles. There is the usual critique of sensationalism in the media, but there is also the complaint that coverage is too conventional, orthodox, careful, and even prim.

The charge of sensationalism is a familiar one and too sweeping to analyze here in any detail. It is related to the competitive nature of journalism, particularly in a democratic free-enterprise society. Journalists compete for television or radio time and newspaper space within their own organizations, while their various information enterprises compete for attention in the marketplace of ideas at the center of our "information society." This system places high value on novelty and significance, as well as on the ability to entertain an audience while informing it. These influences have shaped reporting about medicine and health since 1690 when the first issue of the first newspaper in what is now the United States reported that "epidemical fevers and Agues very common, in some parts of the Country" (quoted in Krieghbaum, 1984, p. 50). Ever since, newspapers have tended to report science and medicine as a series of breakthroughs and epidemics. But at least we no longer have to cope with deliberate hoaxes such as the one that the *New York Sun* published on August 25, 1835, when it claimed that a European astronomer had discovered 4-foot-tall yellowish humanoid creatures on the moon. This was in the days before telegraphs, and the *Sun's* circulation boomed while rival newspapers waited for confirmation or denial to reach them from Europe (Krieghbaum, 1984).

The accusation of journalistic conservatism, though less common, is perhaps equally significant. One version of it was given by Dorothy Nelkin (1987) in her book *Selling Science: How the Press Covers Science and Technology,* which I confess I haven't read. A review of this book by freelance journalist Robert Anderson (1987) quotes her as observing that science journalists tend to be apolitical, to dissociate science from politics, to revere their subject matter, to espouse a norm of objectivity borrowed from 19th-century science, and generally to "identify more closely with their subject and their sources than do journalists in many other fields" (quoted in Anderson, 1987, p. 58). The reviewer notes that "this identification is an ironic one, given the ambivalent if not adversarial attitude scientists manifest toward their journalist counterparts" (Anderson, 1987, p. 60).

Different Worldviews

The tendency of reporters to cover scientists and doctors as if they were 19th-century geniuses working alone in isolated laboratories explains one of the most persistent failures of medical journalism: that it provides its audience with little awareness of the world in which scientists operate. This is particularly true, and perhaps particularly tragic, in the case of medical researchers, especially those in the field of primary care.

Another criticism of medical journalism is that it fails to provide "mobilizing information" that might help people to adopt good health behavior. A study of health reporting in Britain (Kristiansen & Harding, 1984) found that the physiology of illness was reported far more often than the physiology of health; that the press rarely mentioned causes of addictions; that it failed to cite incidence statistics; and that it did not usually mention types of treatment, let alone advocate methods. This was particularly evident when medical reporting was compared with journalism about environmental issues.

The same sort of conclusions were reached by American researchers regarding newspaper coverage of cancer (Freimuth, Greenberg, DeWitt, & Romano, 1984). Sampling news stories from the 50 largest daily newspapers in the United States in 1980, these researchers found that newspapers rarely provided "information on the topics of prevention, risks, detection, and the treatment of cancer, information considered vital to individuals' ability to understand and take action concerning the disease" (Freimuth et al., 1984, p. 67).

In the articles that I surveyed, these criticisms are illustrated by many examples of inadequate reporting of science and medicine in recent decades. The coverage of AIDS predictably draws the most comment. Researchers frequently cite the media's slow response to the AIDS crisis as an example of its narrow definition of news and its conservatism. Because AIDS in the early 1980s was believed to be a disease limited to homosexuals and drug addicts, news media were late in alerting the general public to its dangers; because alerting the public required straightforward descriptions of homosexual activities including anal intercourse, the mass media were unable to bring themselves to the point of doing this until 1985 when the disease already had made swift advances. This narrow, conservative, and prudish definition of acceptable or marketable news deprived many people of information that might have saved their lives.

So we can see that the failure of the media to adequately cover science, medicine, and health issues directly affects the ability of individuals to protect themselves from disease and to support institutional changes that would enable society to improve the systems that promote and protect our well-being. The current confused public debate about health care, specifically the government's response to crises created by rising expectations and static or shrinking resources, has to be seen in part to be a result of this failure.

I would like to mention briefly that our own Graduate School of Journalism is currently involving itself in this problem. With the encouragement of the Pharmaceutical Manufacturers' Association of Canada, and optimistically with the future support of other groups, we have just launched an elective course for our students in medical journalism. We have been fortunate in acquiring one of our distinguished alumni to give this course, in the person of Marilyn Dunlop, the *Toronto Star's* awarding-winning medical journalist for many years. This is the first step toward offering short courses on medical and health issues for working journalists along the lines of those that we already offer in law, economics, and environmental issues. We are proud to be the only Canadian journalism school offering such a portfolio of professional development courses to working journalists and are delighted to add medical journalism to this group.

Finally, a postscript. I would like to make a brief reference to Dr. Ian McWhinney's introduction to *Primary Care Research: Traditional and Innovative Approaches,* Volume One in this series. I was particularly struck by his broad definition of primary care research as he looked ahead to the next 20 years and by his attempt to escape from what I would regard as a narrowly scientific definition of research and to describe a broad reform of the many systems that affect primary care. If this bold attempt is to succeed, it will certainly require careful observation, interpretation, and encouragement by journalists who are also capable of surmounting the old practices and orthodoxies of their craft.

References

Anderson, R. (1987). The credulous and the complacent—A review. *Columbia Journalism Review, 26*(3), 58-60.

Bostian, L. R., & Byrne, T. E. (1984). Comprehension of styles in science writing. *Journalism Quarterly, 61*(3), 676-678.

Calder, I. (1993). *How the* National Enquirer *changed the face of North American journalism.* Lecture reprinted by the Graduate School of Journalism, The University of Western Ontario, London, Ontario.

Dunwoody, S. (1974). *Ethical problems in science writing.* Unpublished manuscript, Temple University, Philadelphia.

Dunwoody, S., & Ryan, M. (1983). Public information persons as mediators between scientists and journalists. *Journalism Quarterly, 60*(4), 647-656.

Dunwoody, S., & Ryan, M. (1985). Scientific barriers to the popularization of science in the mass media. *Journal of Communication, 35*(1), 26-42.

Falk, D. (1991, April). Showtime for science. *Ryerson Review of Journalism,* pp. 46-51.

Freimuth, V. S., Greenberg, R. H., DeWitt, J., & Romano, R. M. (1984). Covering cancer: Newspapers and the public interest. *Journal of Communication, 34*(1), 62-73.

Hallihan, P. (1988). Science reporting accuracy on health topics in the *National Enquirer* and the *Star. Essays in Journalism* (Graduate School of Journalism, The University of Western Ontario), pp. 49-72.

Hinkle, G., & Elliott, W. R. (1989). Science coverage in three newspapers and three supermarket tabloids. *Journalism Quarterly, 66*(2), 353-358.

Johnson, J. D., & Meishcke, H. (1992). Mass media channels—Women's evaluations for cancer-related information. *Newspaper Research Journal, 13*(1 & 2), 146-159.

Krieghbaum, H. (1984). From agues to AIDs. *The Quill, 72*(10), 50-55, 61.

Kristiansen, C. M., & Harding, C. M. (1984). Mobilization of health behaviour by the press in Britain. *Journalism Quarterly, 16*(2), 364-370.

Moore, B., & Singletary, M. (1985). Scientific sources' perceptions of network news accuracy. *Journalism Quarterly, 62*(4), 816-823.

Nelkin, D. (1987). *Selling science: How the press covers science and technology.* New York: Freeman.

Turow, J., & Coe, L. (1985). Curing television's ills: The portrayal of health care. *Journal of Communication, 35*(4), 36-51.

Zimmerman, M. (1988). Many editors ignorant of basic science facts. *American Society of Newspaper Editors Bulletin, 703,* 31.

7 Guidelines for the Dissemination of New Information Discovered by Researchers

PETER G. NORTON
EARL V. DUNN
JOHN BAIN
RICHARD BIRTWHISTLE
DAVID A. DAVIS
CAROL P. HERBERT
JACQUES LEMELIN
ERIC M. MESLIN
YVES TALBOT
MARJORIE L. WOOD

During the planning for the "Foundations of Primary Care Research" conference held in Toronto, Canada, in February 1993, it became apparent that there were no standards or guidelines for the dissemination of research results in primary care. The five editors of the conference proceedings accordingly decided that this volume should contain an answer to the question, "What are the guidelines for the dissemination of new information discovered by primary care researchers?" On reflection the question focused on an examination of the responsibilities of primary care researchers for dissemination of their own findings.

Such guidelines are now necessary for several reasons: Researchers are facing new pressures from the public to ensure that findings are released quickly and with approval of consumers; the development of meta-analysis for combining results of multiple studies has raised concern about the lack of dissemination of negative results and the resulting systematic bias in the summary studies; and there are increasing concerns about fraudulent research and the dissemination of misinformation.

These issues have recently been addressed by a number of authors: Dickerson (1990) has reviewed the issues related to meta-analysis, and Levy, Kjellstrom, Forget, Jones, and Pollier (1992) demonstrated in a recent study that even researchers working in the same area are often unaware of each others' work and results. One important reason that some projects do not receive peer-reviewed funding could be due to their proposals containing unclear or uncertain plans for utilization and dissemination of the findings (Thomas & Lawrence, 1990). One recent attempt to enhance the dissemination of written material has been the development of the concept of more formal "structured abstracts" (Haynes, Mulrow, Huth, Altman, & Gardner, 1990) to help practitioners and researchers better access and more efficiently review the rapidly expanding body of new medical information.

Prior to the "Foundations" conference, the organizers assembled a panel of primary care researchers to address the need and implications of dissemination in primary care research and to prepare a draft set of guidelines. The panel included representatives from academic departments of family medicine in Canada and the United Kingdom, researchers in primary care, basic science and clinical science; the editor of a medical journal; and a bioethicist. The panel comprised the authors of this chapter. A modified Delphi technique (Linstone & Turoff, 1975) was employed in an attempt to achieve a number of consensus statements that could then be presented to the international audience of primary care researchers who were scheduled to meet at the conference.

This chapter outlines the process used to develop the consensus statements and presents details of the proposed guidelines. We remind the reader that guidelines are not the same as standards, but simply act as guideposts and should be followed when appropriate. Nonetheless, when deviating from a guideline one should be able to justify this action to oneself, one's peers, and other stakeholders.

The Process

Two of this book's editors (PGN & EVD) agreed to facilitate the guidelines development process. In an extensive review of the primary care literature, including a Medline search using as key words the terms *researcher* or *research, dissemination,* and *guidelines* or *standards,* they were unable to identify any statement of guidelines for researchers, primary care or otherwise, with respect to the dissemination of one's own discoveries. The search did, however, produce 81 citations related to research dissemination; these papers were reviewed and the content used to produce a preliminary set of statements. These statements were reviewed first by the five editors and then circulated to our expert panel.

Following this first stage, a set of consensus statements, a preliminary responsibility table (a table that depicted consumers of new research knowledge in one dimension and possible disseminators in the other), and a page for open-ended comments were presented to the panel with the following instructions:

This process will attempt to establish consensus guidelines to address the question "What are the guidelines for the dissemination of new information discovered by primary care researchers?" *Clearly there are issues with respect to accuracy, timing, format, etc., that others involved in the dissemination of research results must address, but in what follows we are considering the responsibilities of the researcher(s) only.*

For the consensus statements, the panel members were requested to rate each statement using two Likert scales, as follows:

For each of the following statements please indicate if you agree or disagree on a 5-point scale with −2 meaning strongly disagree, −1 meaning disagree, 0 being neutral, 1 meaning agree and 2 meaning strongly agree. Then assign an importance score from 1 to 5 to each statement. Importance means the relevance of the statement as a principle for primary care researchers. Note that agreement and importance are independent. That is, you can, for example, consider a statement to be very important but in a very negative sense and thus give it a very important score and at the same time disagree strongly. 1 will mean very unimportant, 2 unimportant, 3 undecided/neutral, 4 important and 5 very important.

Thus there were two Likert scales for each statement, one for agreement and one for importance.

For the responsibility table the instructions were:

> In this section there is a table. Across the top are various constituencies to whom research findings might be disseminated. Down the side are the various participants in the dissemination process. Please fill in the following chart with the numbers 0 to 5. Here 0 means the participant in that row *is not at all responsible* to disseminate to the group in that column and 5 means the player *is very responsible*. Thus, if the score in the top left-hand box is zero it means that the research team is not at all responsible to disseminate findings to the funding sources.

The panel had to respond very expeditiously, so fax communication was used. Using standard Delphi methods, each round took less than a week. By the end of the second round there was clear consensus on many of the statements and two new ones had been added. A teleconference was then held to examine the results and consider the areas of major disagreement. Finally, two further Delphi rounds were undertaken with the more than 100 participants who attended the conference; these rounds resulted in some further changes.

The next section presents those statements that were agreed or not agreed upon, and shows the final version of the responsibility table.

Results

At the end of the process, a number of statements were agreed upon (by more than 80% of the final conference respondents, with no strong disagreement) as important guidelines for primary care researchers with respect to the dissemination of new knowledge that they had discovered. These statements are presented in Table 7.1. Table 7.2 shows the two statements that were discarded as unacceptable by the group during the various stages of the Delphi process. Of more interest are those statements where no consensus was reached (in fact, several of these caused considerable heated discussion). These are presented in Table 7.3.

The responsibilities chart is presented in Table 7.4 and indicates the final consensus as to whether the groups represented by the

Table 7.1 Agreed-Upon Statements

♦ Researchers conducting studies with public funding must ensure the dissemination of their findings.

♦ If a study is funded from a private source there is as much responsibility for the dissemination of findings as if public funding were involved.

♦ It is never responsible to disseminate information known to be false.

♦ Information that is disseminated must be understandable and not obscure the clinical significance of the new information.

♦ Any report of the research findings must acknowledge and transmit relevant previous findings (e.g., other investigators' findings, whether supportive or not).

♦ All contributions and help must be acknowledged through authorship or otherwise.

♦ Researchers have responsibility for the timing of dissemination through the public media.

♦ All disseminated results must credit all funding sources.

♦ If a researcher chooses to disseminate only part of the findings, then these must be consistent with the total findings. This partial disclosure must not in any way be fraudulent or misleading.

♦ When the results are rejected for dissemination by several sources, if the researcher is committed to the findings, then continued efforts to disseminate are warranted.

Table 7.2 Statements Rejected by Consensus

♦ Personal gratification and academic advancement are important reasons for dissemination.

♦ Any research results that the researcher chooses to disseminate must be acceptable to the population from which the study sample was drawn.

Table 7.3 Statement Where There Was No Consensus

♦ It is essential that knowledge achieved through research be disseminated for its own sake.

♦ It is responsible not to disseminate in certain cases (e.g., studies with low power).

♦ The results of research must initially be disseminated only through peer-reviewed sources.

rows should have responsibility for the dissemination of new primary care research information to the constituencies represented by the columns. Each box displays either Y for yes, N for no, or ? for no agreement. For example, the Y in the first box indicates that there was consensus that a research team has responsibility to disseminate findings to its funders.

Discussion

The material presented above is, at most, the first step in the development of guidelines to help primary care researchers better understand their obligations with respect to the dissemination of their findings and is presented to stimulate discussion and encourage further attempts to outline the academic, ethical, and professional responsibilities involved.

The statements presented in Table 7.1 were for the most part agreed upon by all who participated. Only two generated significant discussion: (a) that all contributions and help must be acknowledged through authorship or otherwise, and (b) that researchers have responsibility for the timing of dissemination through the public media. In the first of these, the discussion centered around how inclusive the statement should be—would, for example, a casual discussion a year before funding was achieved constitute "help" for the purposes of this guideline? The groups agreed with the spirit of the statement, but also felt that it should be rewritten to reflect this concern. In the second case there was consensus that this principle was desirable but frequently not achievable.

The statements in Table 7.2 were those that were rejected. There was full consensus on rejecting the first, but with the second (relating to the acceptability of results) a committed minority felt that this statement should have been included as a guideline. As one reason for their concern, this group referred to the harm that has befallen certain populations in the past as a result of research findings (e.g., First Nations populations) and also felt that this statement realistically reflects the mood of the public as consumerism becomes a stronger force in medical research.

The statements in Table 7.3 generated disagreement and the most discussion. On the question of whether it is essential that knowledge achieved through research be disseminated for its own sake, one side took the viewpoint that the public has a right to know what research information is available and that information availability is distinct from the ability of an audience to accept or reject such information. For the other side, the argument focused on the possible harm that can and has resulted from new knowledge (nuclear weapons and genetic engineering were cited as examples).

On the question of whether it is responsible not to disseminate in certain cases (e.g., studies with low power), those in agreement were concerned about systematic bias in the literature if not all information is available, whereas the other side noted the effect that results of low power can have when disseminated to the public, who may not appreciate the significant possibility of error.

Finally, regarding whether the results of research must initially be disseminated only through peer-reviewed sources, some of the disagreement centered around what is meant by "results." If we consider the "Ingelfinger Rule" (Relman, 1981), then this means final results only. During the course of research, however, especially in primary care settings where many collaborators are involved (e.g., network research), ongoing communication with the team and to the subjects may increase compliance and recruitment. When analyzed and interpreted data are presented that may have an impact on the health care system, peer review becomes an important if not essential step.

The responsibility table (Table 7.4) contains several interesting results. First, editors of journals will be interested to learn that our consensus group considers that their only clear responsibility is to inform practitioners. Recently Haynes (1990) examined peer-reviewed journals from this perspective and concluded that editors "sometimes impede the dissemination of validated advances to practitioners" (p. 724). He goes on to suggest changes that might help address this problem.

Second, research teams should ponder their responsibilities to their subjects, because they were the only ones felt to be responsible for dissemination to this group. In addition, policy makers, professional bodies, and regulatory groups have, according to our panel, a strong responsibility to disseminate to practitioners and the public. We would hope that they would apprise themselves of the opinions we have uncovered here and act accordingly; perhaps

Table 7.4 Responsibilities for Dissemination

To → By ↓	Funders	Research Peers	Practitioners	Policy Makers & Regulatory Bodies**	Research Subjects	Public
Research Team	Y	Y	Y	?	Y	?
Academics	?	Y	Y	Y	?	?
Editors of Journals	N	?	Y	?	N	?
Professional Bodies*	?	?	Y	Y	?	Y
Public Media	?	N	?	?	?	Y
Policy Makers	?	?	Y	Y	N	Y
Regulatory Bodies**	?	?	Y	Y	N	Y

NOTES: Y = Agreement that dissemination should be done
N = Agreement that dissemination should not be done
? = No consensus
* e.g., the Royal College of Physicians and Surgeons of Canada
** e.g., licensing bodies

it is the responsibility of the research community to draw the attention of these groups to the findings of our process.

In summary, we have begun to look systematically at the responsibilities and roles around dissemination of research information and hope that our efforts will stimulate continued contemplation and discussion around this area.

References

Dickerson, K. (1990). The existence of publication bias and risk factors for its occurrence. *Journal of the American Medical Association, 263*(10), 1385-1389.

Haynes, R. B. (1990). Loose connections between peer-reviewed clinical journals and clinical practice. *Annals of Internal Medicine, 113*(9), 724-728.

Haynes, R. B., Mulrow, C. D., Huth, E. J., Altman, D. G., & Gardner, M. J. (1990). More informative abstracts revisited. *Annals of Internal Medicine, 113*(1), 69-76.

Levy, B. S., Kjellstrom, T., Forget, G., Jones, M. R., & Pollier, L. (1992). Ongoing research in occupational health and environmental epidemiology in developing countries. *Archives of Environmental Health, 47*(3), 231-235.

Linstone, H. A., & Turoff, M. (Eds.). (1975). *The Delphi method—Techniques and applications.* Reading, MA: Addison-Wesley.

Relman, A. S. (1981). The Ingelfinger rule. *New England Journal of Medicine, 305*(14), 824-826.

Thomas, J. P., & Lawrence, T. S. (1990). Common deficiencies of NIDRR research applications. *American Journal of Physical Medicine and Rehabilitation, 60*(2), 73-76.

PART II

Methodology Issues

8 How to Do Research on Dissemination

PENNY JENNETT

The dissemination process is dynamic and complex, whether considered from the perspective of the individual or the organization. Individuals become aware of an idea, assess its value, and decide either to adopt or reject it. If adoption is chosen, the processes of implementation and confirmation begin. Change does not take place without attention to need, readiness, compatibility, trialability, adaptability, and norms. Similarly, before deciding to adopt an idea, organizations collect information, conceptualize, and plan. Implementation involves a further series of events termed as redefining, restructuring, clarifying, and scrutinizing (Rogers, 1983).

Given the involved, complicated, and fluid nature of the dissemination process itself, it is not surprising that research specific to it would be both challenging and unique. Indeed, Rogers (1983) proposes that this research involves the study of human behavior centered around nine scientific disciplines: anthropology, early sociology, rural sociology, education, public health and medical sociology, communications, marketing, geography, and general sociology. As well, investigations on dissemination often must employ well-controlled, rigorous epidemiologic methods hand in hand with qualitative approaches requiring flexibility and reframing. In addition, such studies often unfold under uncontrolled conditions at both the practice and policy levels.

Dissemination research activities can be greatly enhanced if four prerequisites are in place: a clear definition of the dissemination process, an openness to research approaches beyond conventional methods, an awareness and informed appreciation for previous dissemination work, and a well-thought-out, detailed research plan. These points will be briefly addressed in turn.

First, regarding a definition, one must explicitly articulate an appropriate definition for one's investigations before initiating related research activities. Selecting which step(s) within the dissemination process to investigate, along with the appropriate process and outcome measures, can only begin with a clear understanding of the term itself. Two established definitions are offered for the reader, one presented in 1992 by the Agency for Health Care Policy and Research (AHCPR), U.S. Department of Health and Human Services, and another by Rogers (1983). The AHCPR defines *dissemination* as "the process through which target groups become aware of, receive, accept, and utilize disseminated information"; its goal being the improvement of "patient care, patient outcomes, and quality of life" (p. 2). Rogers uses the terms *diffusion* and *dissemination* interchangeably to refer to both the intended and unintended dispersion of novel information. He states diffusion to be "the process by which an innovation is communicated through certain channels over time among the members of a social system" (p. 5).

Regarding openness, McWhinney (1991) alerts investigators wishing to engage in dissemination research of the need to value different research approaches and methods. He indicates that a skilled sensitivity to conventional investigative approaches, along with a genuine value for context, meaning, and understanding, is required. The inquiry process is interactive rather than passive. Therefore, the expectations of more traditional research perspectives, that is, control, prediction, generalizability, and causality, may be somewhat limiting.

Regarding awareness, researchers must be familiar with the growing body of literature on dissemination. Information transfer and utilization is a dynamic, fluid, and iterative process that is dependent upon a complex entwining of individual psychological influences, professional and societal norms, and organizational/environmental contexts (Fox, 1991; Fox, Mazmanian, & Putnam, 1989; Nowlen, 1988; see also Chapters 1 and 2 in this volume). Forces that facilitate and impede change play a role, as do principles and ideas specific to stages of change; readiness to change; formal as well as informal communication networks; and opinion leaders, change agents, and educational influentials (Geertsma,

Parker, & Whitbourne, 1982; Greer, 1988; Hiss, MacDonald, & Davis, 1978; Lewin, 1951; Lomas, 1991; Lomas et al., 1988; Lomas et al., 1989; Moore-West, Northup, Skipper, & Teaf, 1984; Rogers, 1983; Stross & Harlan, 1981; Wackman, Miller, & Nunnaly, 1976; Weinberg, Ullian, Richards, & Cooper, 1981; Williams & Boulton, 1988). Successful dissemination strategies are recognized as incorporating an appreciation of the context; an adequately detailed assessment of needs based on practice links; and enabling, predisposing, and reinforcing strategies (Davis, Thomson, Oxman, & Haynes, 1992; see also Chapter 11 in this volume). Lomas (Chapter 1, this volume) summarizes the issues by outlining alternative theoretical perspectives that are related to the social influence model, the diffusion of innovation literature, adult learning theory, and marketing approaches.

Finally, a rigorous planning process is critical to meaningful and successful research activities. Van de Ven and Rogers (1988) specify four requirements that should be in place to undertake dissemination research. Specifically, they suggest that investigators must have a clear sense of the concepts being studied, systematic methods for observing change over time, methods for representing process patterns, and theory to make sense of the process. In addition, Metcalfe (1992) outlines specific issues that are important to determine in the planning stage. He states that the specific clinical activities to be evaluated, the number of examples required, the frequency of measurement, who is to gather and analyze data, the outcomes to be assessed, and the required resources and costs are all items to be clearly defined. As well, there are frequently several audiences involved in the area of dissemination; for example, practitioners, patients, professional bodies, practice organizations, health care systems, policy makers, researchers, and the media. Each of these groups possesses different perspectives associated with the transfer and utilization of information. All relevant parties who are designated as part of the investigative team should be involved in the planning phase to insure appropriate contextual viewpoints.

Research Steps

There are nine classic steps in the dissemination research process. Quality and attention to standards at all phases are required (Dunn, 1991; Kuzel & Like, 1991).

STEP 1: REVIEWING THE LITERATURE

A careful and critical review of the literature is imperative to permit a clear statement of purpose and to choose the optimal theoretical and methodological approaches for a study. Key references that focus on relevant issues should be read with care and earmarked for the research planning and writing stages. In the critique of previous studies, particular notations should be made of the dissemination aspect being examined; the type of innovation; the unit of analysis; the data collection and analysis methods; and the major findings, recommendations, and limitations.

STEP 2: DEFINING AND REFINING QUESTIONS

Stewart (1992) and Bordage (1989) emphasize the central importance of the research question. The former states that it provides the study's foundation; the latter designates it as the backbone.

Howie (1991) outlines characteristics of a good research question as follows. It must be important, relevant, interesting, challenging, and stated simply. Data required to study the questions must be accessible. Questions should be based upon needs, experience, and past research. Specific to the dissemination field, researchers must be clear as to whether they are trying to understand and explain aspects of the dissemination process, generate or test hypotheses, determine appropriate intervention processes, compare different methods of dissemination, describe and evaluate the process, and/or predict. They must decide if they wish to assess whether audiences have become informed, made decisions, changed behavior, and/or improved quality care—in short, the research focus must be clear as to which components of the dissemination process and which outcomes are being addressed.

STEP 3: DESCRIBING STUDY CONTEXT AND VARIABLES

The context in which the study is to be conducted must be clearly delineated to ensure a quality research plan and design, as well as an appropriate interpretation of findings. All variables (independent and dependent) must be defined for the researchers, the readers, and the funding sources. Individual, social, and communication variables should be considered. Depending upon the study question, process (style of care) and/or health care outcome measures may be most appropriate for study. Metcalfe (1992) provides guidance regarding outcomes in General Practice, and offers definitions for three components of quality that can be considered in such research—effectiveness, efficiency, and patient satisfaction.

STEP 4: RESEARCH DESIGN AND METHODS

The study design provides the blueprint for the activity (Stewart, 1992), and as such is central to quality investigation. Dissemination research may involve descriptive (practice audits, surveys, case reports), explanatory or analytic, qualitative, or a combination of study designs. A composite of quantitative and qualitative approaches is seen by some as optimal (Helman, 1991; Janes, Stall, & Gifford, 1986; Tudiver et al., 1991). In particular, Dunn (1991) provides standards for analytic studies (cross-sectional, case control, cohort, and randomized and nonrandomized controlled trials); Kuzel and Like (1991) provide them for qualitative work. Longitudinal, prospective, multidisciplinary, and collaborative perspectives are worthy of consideration. For example, for tracing the sequential nature of information adoption within a system, Rogers (1983) specifically recommends field experiments, longitudinal panel studies, archival records, and case studies.

A sampling technique and appropriate study population are required. Attention to sample size factors in both qualitative and quantitative research approaches is required. For quantitative consideration, Østbye (1992) provides insightful guidance regarding population and sampling units. The strengths and weaknesses associated with office-based, workplace, volunteer, community, random, cluster, and stratified samplings are offered. He reviews the importance of delineating population factors such as content, extent, and time, as well as the importance of distinct sampling units. Characteristics of representative sampling and generalizability are outlined.

If embarking on qualitative research, researchers would be well advised to reflect on Kuzel's (1992) article when considering sampling factors. Such issues as what to sample, how to sample, features of sampling, and a sampling typology are provided in this work. Context is central to qualitative research: whereas generalizability and representativeness, are challenged.

Data collection methods and data sources require careful selection. Informed choices regarding which information collection tools to adopt, given the research question posed, are vital to the success of any project. The chosen measurement tools are "the bricks, mortar, hammers, and lathe. Without these even the most elegantly designed structures do not rise above the foundation" (Stewart, 1992, pp. xv-xvii). A difficult but critical issue is whether investigators adopt tools that have been previously applied or construct new ones. The former may sacrifice some construct and content validity; the latter requires substantial expertise, time, and resources to optimize quality and reliability (Tudiver & Ferris, 1992).

Epidemiological as well as ethnographic data collection methods are often required. Particularly for the former, Wilkin (1992) provides an overview of criteria to consider when determining optimal measurement instruments. Chosen tools must be able to assess what is to be measured, be applied in a standardized manner, and be appropriate for the level of measurement required. Reliability, validity, and responsiveness are necessary instrument characteristics, as are objectivity and precision. On the other hand, Zyzanski (1992) provides valuable guidelines specific to qualitative information-gathering methods. Here, such terms as *data credibility, dependability,* and *confirmability* often replace *reliability* and *validity.* Triangulation methods and reflection are in place to support such characteristics and provide evidence for information trustworthiness.

Norr (Chapter 9, this volume) provides a comprehensive summary of qualitative and quantitative methods for gathering data, along with their strengths and weaknesses and when they might best be used. In addition, previous volumes in this series (Volumes 2 and 3) are particularly valuable resources for decision making in this area. All chosen data collection instruments should be pilot-tested and appropriately revised prior to the onset of the main study.

The context in which the instruments are to be applied is a central factor in tool selection. When making instrument choices, one must always consider the feasibility of information collection in this context, along with issues of accessibility, ownership, and confidentiality. Data sources must be accessible and credible if the quality of information collected is to be defended and meaningfully interpreted. Both primary and secondary sources can often be used. Given the contextual nature of the research, investigators should be prepared for indirect and unintended benefits and barriers, as well as for the planned measures (Chapter 9, this volume). Rogers (1983) defines three types of consequences: desirable versus undesirable, direct versus indirect, and anticipated versus unanticipated.

Researchers should always keep in mind that each selected tool (or combination of tools) has its unique strengths and weaknesses. Snapshot or one-time surveys, popular in earlier research, are valued for the information they can provide, but are now recognized as being limited specific to both the time linkages between independent and dependent variables, as well as causality.

Appropriate data analysis techniques are fundamental to quality work. A careful descriptive review of all collected data is wise as a first step. Then, depending upon the selected research questions, either quantitative and/or qualitative analyses may be appropriate. Quantitative analysis methods involving both descriptive and inferential (univariate and multivariate) techniques may be required. More complex inferential data analyses should always be verified with a qualified biostatistician. With respect to qualitative techniques, informed guidelines and software packages are now available to assist researchers. The content and text analysis of narratives, along with many qualitative terms such as *saturation* and *themes* require understanding in order for accurate qualitative analyses to proceed (Crabtree & Miller, 1992).

The data analysis approaches must always be chosen to match the questions being posed and must be appropriate to the assumptions in place. For researchers selecting a combination quantitative analysis/qualitative analysis approach, the iterative nature of the second must always be kept in mind.

STEP 5: ASSESSING RESOURCES REQUIRED,
OUTLINING A BUDGET, AND SPECIFYING
A TIME FRAME FOR RESEARCH ACTIVITIES

Accurately determining or estimating the resources required to conduct a research project is a skill that often evolves through experience. For investigators who are fairly new to dissemination research, a good rule of thumb is to discuss this step with colleagues carrying out similar work. Underestimating resources can result in having either to terminate a project midway or before results can be shared with colleagues.

A careful outline of resource and budgetary needs is also a prerequisite for approaching potential funding sources. As dissemination research often involves partnerships, funding may require collaboration with industry, community, or government. Both public and private sectors may be involved. Either granting or contracting arrangements, or both, may be appropriate.

Estimating a time and work schedule for the research activities is essential for accurate budget predictions. For this task, careful work in Steps 1 through 4 pays off. All the insights and directions that surface during these steps contribute to informed estimates of resource requirements.

STEP 6: ETHICAL ISSUES

Dissemination research, like all primary care investigations, requires approval by an Ethics Review Board. As several stakeholders are usually collaboratively involved, issues of ownership, release of information, confidentiality, and access need to be worked out prior to the initiation of the research. The timing for release of findings requires thought and collaborative scholarly decision making. Informed-consent forms for all participating subjects should be in place.

STEP 7: PRESENTING DATA

Tables, graphs, figures, and charts are always helpful in displaying descriptive data. Classical ways of presenting univariate and multivariate results are acceptable if these forms of quantitative analyses have been used. If qualitative approaches to data analyses have been adopted, Morse (Chapter 5, this volume) provides an excellent overview of how to display such data using recognized standards, including diagramming, modeling, and use of tables.

STEP 8: INTERPRETING DATA AND PRESENTING
A DISCUSSION

Deciding on how best to interpret the data involves returning to the partnership of stakeholders who comprise the investigators. Each should be encouraged to provide a perspective on the assembled results. Data interpretation should be limited to members of the research team.

Further, to facilitate informed data interpretation, each study result should be revisited to reflect on what it means in the context of the problem being studied and the literature reviewed. What insights or additional knowledge the study has provided to the field should be noted, along with the issues requiring further study and the study's limitations.

STEP 9: WRITING UP AND SHARING THE FINDINGS

Because research in dissemination is very complex and fairly new, it is critical that its findings and implications be shared with colleagues embarking upon similar types of endeavors. Writing up results for both presentation and publication forums is therefore important. Bordage (1989) provides an excellent classic overview for researchers preparing work for publication, including a checklist that is an effective practical tool for achieving publication goals. Morse (Chapter 5, this volume) reviews techniques for effectively disseminating qualitative research results. One of her points is that investigators must target their messages to specific audiences and journals, and when preparing presentations or manuscripts must keep in mind the specific needs of both.

Conclusion

Dissemination research shares a common theme with all other types of research: It demands careful planning to optimize quality, feasibility, and successful completion. Factors that can be helpful in carrying out a successful project include an informed knowledge of previous dissemination work, a firm grasp of which component of the dissemination process is being studied, a clearly defined research question, and a comfort with both traditional and unconventional research approaches.

Much can be found in the published literature that can assist those engaged in dissemination work. Most studies to date have investigated the characteristics and motivations of innovators; the practitioners' readiness to change; the change process within and across individuals, organizations, or social systems; the roles of opinion leaders and change agents; the characteristics and use of dissemination networks; the design of effective dissemination packages; and the consequences of innovations. There have been calls for other types of investigations to further advance the field (Rogers, 1983), in particular, those that either focus on the dissemination process as it unfolds; gather data at multiple points of the process; compare successful and unsuccessful attempts at information transfer and adoption; or examine how innovations are adapted to individuals, groups, and social systems.

The challenges of dissemination research are many; its importance is indisputable. The research questions to be posed and answered are critical to ongoing quality health care delivery and informed policy making. The expertise and resources to conduct meaningful research are now available and responsibility lies heavily among researchers from several disciplines. The continued successful completion of significant and feasible investigative dissemination activities is dependent upon turning to this expertise and to the existing related literature.

References

Agency for Health Care Policy and Research [AHCPR]. (1992). *Annotated bibliography: Information dissemination to health practitioners and policymakers.* Washington, DC: Department of Health and Human Services.

Bordage, G. (1989). Considerations on preparing a paper for publication. *Teaching and Learning in Medicine, 1*(1), 47-52.

Crabtree, B. F., & Miller, W. L. (1992). The analysis of narrative from a long interview. In M. Stewart, F. Tudiver, M. J. Bass, E. V. Dunn, & P. G. Norton (Eds.), *Tools for primary care research* (pp. 209-220). Newbury Park, CA: Sage.

Davis, D. A., Thomson, M. A., Oxman, A. D., & Haynes, R. B. (1992). Evidence for the effectiveness of CME: A review of 50 randomized controlled trials. *Journal of the American Medical Association, 268*(9), 1111-1117.

Dunn, E. V. (1991). Basic standards for analytic studies in primary care research. In P. G. Norton, M. Stewart, F. Tudiver, M. J. Bass, & E. V. Dunn (Eds.),

Primary care research: Traditional and innovative approaches (pp. 78-96). Newbury Park, CA: Sage.

Fox, R. D. (1991). New research agendas for CME: Organizing principles for the study of self-directed curricula for change. *Journal of Continuing Education in the Health Professionals, 11,* 155-167.

Fox, R. D., Mazmanian, P. E., & Putnam, R. W. (1989). *Changing and learning in the lives of physicians.* New York: Praeger.

Geertsma, R. H., Parker, R. C., & Whitbourne, S. K. (1982). How physicians view the process of change in their practice behavior. *Journal of Medical Education, 57,* 752-768.

Greer, A. L. (1988). The state of the art versus the state of the science: The diffusion of new medical technologies into practice. *International Journal of Technology Assessment in Health Care, 4,* 5-26.

Helman, C. G. (1991). Research in primary care: The qualitative approach. In P. G. Norton, M. Stewart, F. Tudiver, M. J. Bass, & E. V. Dunn (Eds.), *Primary care research: Traditional and innovative approaches* (pp. 105-124). Newbury Park, CA: Sage.

Hiss, R. G., MacDonald, R., & Davis, W. K. (1978). Identification of physician educational influentials (EI) in small community hospitals. *Proceedings of the 17th Annual Conference in Medical Education: Association of American Medical Colleges,* New Orleans, LA, pp. 283-288.

Howie, J. G. R. (1991). Refining questions and hypotheses. In P. G. Norton, M. Stewart, F. Tudiver, M. J. Bass, & E. V. Dunn (Eds.), *Primary care research: Traditional and innovative approaches* (pp. 13-25). Newbury Park, CA: Sage.

Janes, C., Stall, R., & Gifford, S. (1986). *Anthropology and epidemiology.* Dordrecht, Holland: Reidel.

Kuzel, A. J. (1992). Sampling in qualitative inquiry. In B. F. Crabtree & W. L. Miller (Eds.), *Doing qualitative research* (pp. 31-44). Newbury Park, CA: Sage.

Kuzel, A. J., & Like, R. C. (1991). Standards of trustworthiness for qualitative studies in primary care. In P. G. Norton, M. Stewart, F. Tudiver, M. J. Bass, & E. V. Dunn (Eds.), *Primary care research: Traditional and innovative approaches* (pp. 138-158). Newbury Park, CA: Sage.

Lewin, K. (1951). *Field theory in social science.* New York: Harper & Row.

Lomas, J. (1991). Words without actions? The production, dissemination and impact of consensus recommendations. *Annual Review of Public Health, 12,* 41-65.

Lomas, J., Anderson, G. M., Dominick-Pierre, K., Vayda, E., Enkin, M. W., & Hannah, W. J. (1989). Do practice guidelines guide practice? The effect of a consensus statement on the practice of physicians. *New England Journal of Medicine, 321*(19), 1306-1311.

Lomas, J. G., Anderson, G. M., Enkin, M., Vayda, E., Roberts, R., & MacKinnon, B. (1988). The role of evidence in the consensus process: Results from a Canadian consensus exercise. *Journal of the American Medical Association, 259*(20), 3001-3005.

McWhinney, I. R. (1991). Primary care research in the next twenty years. In P. G. Norton, M. Stewart, F. Tudiver, M. J. Bass, & E. V. Dunn (Eds.), *Primary care research: Traditional and innovative approaches* (pp. 1-12). Newbury Park, CA: Sage.

Metcalfe, D. (1992). The measurement of outcomes in general practice. In M. Stewart, F. Tudiver, M. J. Bass, E. V. Dunn, & P. G. Norton (Eds.), *Tools for primary care research* (pp. 14-27). Newbury Park, CA: Sage.

Moore-West, M., Northup, D., Skipper, B., & Teaf, D. (1984). Information-seeking behavior among physicians practicing in urban and nonurban areas. *Proceedings of the Twenty-third Annual Conference—Research in Medical Education*, Chicago, pp. 237-242.

Nowlen, P. M. (1988). *A new approach to continuing education for business and the professions.* New York: Collier Macmillan.

Østbye, T. (1992). How to select a sample in primary care research. In M. Stewart, F. Tudiver, M. J. Bass, E. V. Dunn, & P. G. Norton (Eds.), *Tools for primary care research* (pp. 77-85). Newbury Park, CA: Sage.

Rogers, E. M. (1983). *Diffusion of innovations* (3rd ed.). New York: Free Press.

Stewart, M. (1992). Introduction. In M. Stewart, F. Tudiver, M. J. Bass, E. V. Dunn, & P. G. Norton (Eds.), *Tools for primary care research* (pp. xv-xvii). Newbury Park, CA: Sage.

Stross, J. K., & Harlan, W. P. (1981). Dissemination of relevant information on hypertension. *Journal of the American Medical Association, 246,* 360-362.

Tudiver, F., Cushman, R. A., Crabtree, B. F., Miller, W. L., Manca, D. P., & Brown, J. B. (1991). Combining quantitative and qualitative methodologies in primary care: Some examples. In P. G. Norton, M. Stewart, F. Tudiver, M. J. Bass, & E. V. Dunn (Eds.), *Primary care research: Traditional and innovative approaches* (pp. 159-180). Newbury Park, CA: Sage.

Tudiver, F., & Ferris, L. E., (1992). Creating an original measure. In M. Stewart, F. Tudiver, M. J. Bass, E. V. Dunn, & P. G. Norton (Eds.), *Tools for primary care research* (pp. 86-96). Newbury Park, CA: Sage.

Van De Ven, A. H., & Rogers, E. M. (1988). Innovations and organizations: Critical perspectives. *Communication Research, 15*(5), 632-651.

Wackman, D. B., Miller, S., & Nunnaly, E. W. (1976). *Student workbook: Increasing awareness in communication skills.* Minneapolis, MN: Interpersonal Communication Programs.

Weinberg, A. D., Ullian, L., Richards, W. D., & Cooper, P. (1981). Informal advice and information-seeking between physicians. *Journal of Medical Education, 56,* 174-180.

Wilkin, D. (1992). Selecting an instrument to measure the outcomes of health care. In M. Stewart, F. Tudiver, M. J. Bass, E. V. Dunn, & P. G. Norton (Eds.), *Tools for primary care research* (pp. 50-63). Newbury Park, CA: Sage.

Williams, A., & Boulton, M. (1988). Thinking prevention: Concepts and constructs in general practice. In M. Lock & D. R. Gordon (Eds.), *Biomedicine examined* (pp. 227-255). London: Kluwer Academic.

Zyzanski, S. J. (1992). Cutting and pasting new measures for old. In M. Stewart, F. Tudiver, M. J. Bass, E. V. Dunn, & P. G. Norton (Eds.), *Tools for primary care research* (pp. 97-112). Newbury Park, CA: Sage.

9 Using Quantitative and Qualitative Methods to Assess Impact on Practice

KATHLEEN F. NORR

Introducing an innovation sets off a complex process of change that can have both anticipated and unanticipated effects on the setting, the health care providers, and the patients. Initial research establishing the effectiveness of an innovation is usually done in a carefully controlled and favorable environment. As the innovation is adopted in more realistic conditions, it is essential to know whether it continues to be effective and how it is integrated into and affects the health care setting. Negative impacts affecting factors such as work efficiency, morale, or costs, especially if unanticipated, can lead to the abandonment of an otherwise promising innovation.

My own interest in the impact of innovations stems from my involvement in the introduction of mother/infant "rooming-in" at a large public hospital serving the medically indigent. At this time, rooming-in had been widely adopted in hospitals serving predominately middle-class populations, but there were no published studies of its impact for low-income families. My colleagues and I took advantage of this opportunity to examine its effects on maternal attachment (Norr, Roberts, & Freese, 1989; Norr & Roberts, n.d.). We did not think about looking at other impacts such as positive staff reactions, however. Originally, there was considerable opposition to this innovation. The nursing staff was extremely traditional and even required mothers to be in bed when they held their babies, lest they drop them. The nurses also felt that rooming-in would be more work for them. In a few short months, however, they became enthusiastic supporters. They found that once the initial adjustment period passed it was easier and more satisfying to care for mother-infant dyads; seeing the mothers interact with the infants increased staff respect for them and job satisfaction and professionalism increased. Unfortunately the opportunity to document these changes systematically had been lost due to our failure to think beyond the expected impact of the innovation on patient outcomes.

As this example highlights, there is a need for more case studies of change in a single setting and for comparative studies of multiple settings or multiple innovations. The complexity of conducting such research, however, and the lack of strategies for collecting and analyzing relevant information have been barriers to the systematic investigation of these processes. A combination of qualitative and quantitative strategies is essential to monitor many of the impacts of the changes introduced. Recent theoretical and practical advances in the linking of qualitative and quantitative methods have made such research more feasible today. This chapter will present a working model of major factors that may be affected by an innovation, and specific techniques appropriate for assessing change in each of these factors.

Factors Changed by Health Care Innovations

The process of change is not fully predictable, and the unexpected often occurs along the way. Some working model is, however, essential to help the researcher know where to look for change. At the risk of considerable oversimplification, potential changes can be conceptualized as a function of the interaction between the characteristics of the innovation and the characteristics of a health care setting.

FACTORS RELATED TO THE INNOVATION

Innovations can be categorized according to their scope of impact, likely benefits, and likely costs. Scope of impact can be conceptualized as the number of subunits within the setting likely to be affected; innovations affecting more subunits will probably require more effort to initiate and to continue. Greer (1984) found that scope was important in decisions to introduce innovations of new technologies at community hospitals. Hospital administrators were the primary decision makers for wide-scope innovations, but narrow-scope innovations were often decided upon by doctors in that specialty area.

For most innovations, benefits largely accrue to patients and can be measured by the degree of improvement in patient outcomes and by the number of patients who will benefit. Health care settings will have greater commitment to successfully adopting innovations that have clear benefits for patients. There may, however, be greater willingness to work hard to introduce successful innovations that benefit the providers or the setting as well. Potential benefits for providers include increased professional prestige, reduced workload, reduced difficulty of a particular task, and greater income; benefits to the health care setting include new cost-control strategies, simplified administration, computerized reporting of problems and outcomes, and so forth. Dissention and resentments may develop when an innovation benefits some providers but places new burdens on others or when it benefits the setting but burdens the providers.

Costs include financial, physical plant, and organizational costs. The first, usually the best known, refers to the estimated expense of introducing and maintaining the innovation. Physical plant costs refer to space requirements and any renovations, including inconveniences and temporary or permanent loss of space. Organizational costs include training, reorganization of the administrative and caregiving routines and procedures, renegotiation of the relationships between different types of health professionals and/or other staff, and changes in the caregiver-patient relationship.

Where financial and physical plant costs are high, the administrative unit has correspondingly more say in the decision-making process; where they are low, decisions are more fully in the hands of practitioners. In the typical process of making decisions about an innovation, financial and physical plant costs are given a great deal of attention, but organizational costs are not as carefully considered. In part, this reflects greater uncertainty about what these costs will really be, and in part the likelihood that much of the organizational burden of change will fall on sectors of the organization that are less involved in the decision-making process.

The organizational costs of an innovation are highly relevant to practitioners, especially in the area of primary care where innovations less often involve expensive new equipment and procedures, and more often involve improvements in the more labor-intensive aspects of care. Changes in procedures and structures are always a challenge, first to determine what changes will be needed for an innovation and then to introduce these changes smoothly. In any established health care setting the different workers have evolved a specific working relationship, with a division of labor and formal and informal power relationships that some groups and individuals have a vested interest in maintaining. Many innovations require at least some adjustment in those relationships and may threaten the vested interests of one or more groups. Some innovations, such as the introduction of nurse practitioners into a setting, require major changes.

Many innovations do not require any changes in the practitioner-patient relationship; however, when these sorts of changes are required they can be stressful. For example, the introduction of earlier discharge for many types of patients in the hospital has distressed nurses by reducing time for patient teaching and by increasing nurse workload because the average patient is sicker. Practitioners may feel especially challenged when changes reduce their implicit authority relative to clients.

All these organizational costs are disruptive of the smooth operation of a health care setting and there is a built-in bias in many settings to minimize them as much as possible. Innovations in patient care that require major organizational changes for successful implementation are frequently adopted without adequate provision, either because the extent of change required was not anticipated or because the decision makers were not the ones directly affected by the changes. Failure to successfully make the necessary organizational accommodation can lead to rejection of an otherwise beneficial innovation. In Great Britain, Spiegal et al. (1992) have adapted a strategy from corporate management to identify all the interested parties in primary care settings who will be affected by an innovation, and the costs and benefits to each. They then use group meetings to work through these implementation issues and to facilitate the process of innovation.

Patients and their families also may incur costs when an innovation is introduced. For example, earlier discharge from the hospital may burden a family with additional responsibilities and expense, or a change that affects the patient-provider relation may be distressing to both parties. Unfortunately, the costs for patients may not be considered in the implementation process because they often have no formal role in the decision-making process.

FACTORS RELATED TO THE HEALTH CARE SETTING

When workers at a particular health care setting are contemplating a particular innovation, they can examine what has happened in other settings, especially settings similar to their own, where the innovation has been adopted. They can never be exactly sure, however, what will happen in their own unique setting. A simple model of health care includes its context, its specific practices, and its outcomes (see Figure 9.1). The context of care includes the characteristics of the providers, organizational characteristics of the specific health care setting and the larger health care system in which it is located, and the population served.

Helman (1984) discusses the importance of context, and observes that primary care allows providers to have greater awareness of the context than hospital care, especially relevant factors about patients and their lives. Relevant provider characteristics include the mix of types of health professionals and specialties, their personal backgrounds, prior training, and whether their orientation is cosmopolitan or local. A cosmopolitan orientation, including linkage to the profession outside the community and an attempt to stay current, has been found by Rogers (1983) and others to be especially important in identifying which individuals will be most eager to adopt new innovations. Characteristics of the health care setting include the type of facility (e.g., private family practice or a community hospital); the larger service delivery model of the particular system (e.g., a national health service, a for-profit system serving predominately privately insured patients, or a municipal public facility serving the poor); and the economic pressures and resources. Characteristics of the population served include their social and economic mix, their culture and language, and their levels of health knowledge and demands for service. The size and diversity of the population are also rele-

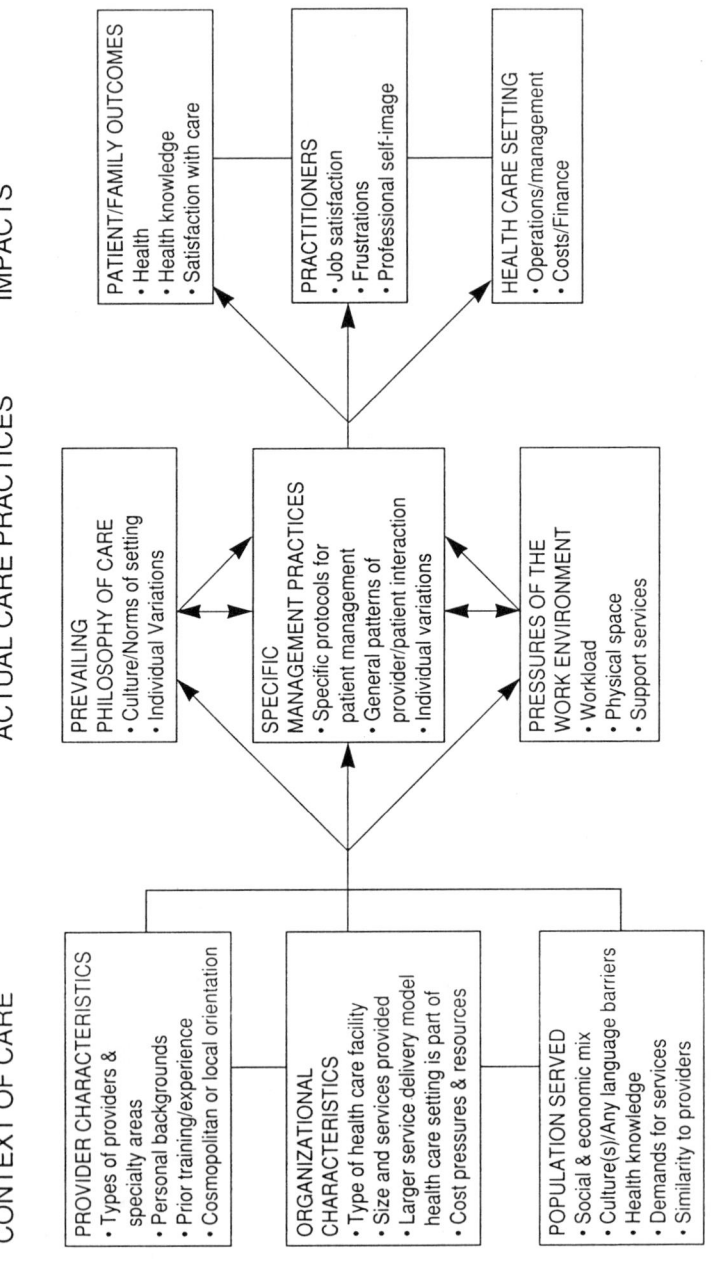

Figure 9.1. Changing Health Care Practices: A Theoretical Framework

CONTEXT OF CARE

PROVIDER CHARACTERISTICS
• Types of providers & specialty areas
• Personal backgrounds
• Prior training/experience
• Cosmopolitan or local orientation

ORGANIZATIONAL CHARACTERISTICS
• Type of health care facility
• Size and services provided
• Larger service delivery model health care setting is part of
• Cost pressures & resources

POPULATION SERVED
• Social & economic mix
• Culture(s)/Any language barriers
• Health knowledge
• Demands for services
• Similarity to providers

ACTUAL CARE PRACTICES

PREVAILING PHILOSOPHY OF CARE
• Culture/Norms of setting
• Individual Variations

SPECIFIC MANAGEMENT PRACTICES
• Specific protocols for patient management
• General patterns of provider/patient interaction
• Individual variations

PRESSURES OF THE WORK ENVIRONMENT
• Workload
• Physical space
• Support services

IMPACTS

PATIENT/FAMILY OUTCOMES
• Health
• Health knowledge
• Satisfaction with care

PRACTITIONERS
• Job satisfaction
• Frustrations
• Professional self-image

HEALTH CARE SETTING
• Operations/management
• Costs/Finance

114

vant, as well as the degree of social, economic, cultural, and language similarity or difference between them and the care providers.

The actual care practices include the culture or prevailing philosophy of the setting, pressure of the work environment, and the specific health management practices that result from these. In every health care setting, a prevailing philosophy of practice gradually develops out of the interaction of the characteristics of the practitioners, the setting, and the population served. This philosophy is a complex set of collective norms and values about how practitioners and patients should interact, what patients are like, what a "good practitioner" and a "good patient" are, and what the health care setting's role is. The fact that these norms are not written down and may seldom be discussed does not lessen their importance in shaping patient care. Equally important are the constraining factors in the environment, such as patient load; presence or absence of equipment, supplies, and support services; and the physical space. Perhaps the most critical set of factors is the actual care practices, including usual protocols and procedures followed for different symptoms and diagnoses, the manner in which patients are treated, and the extent and content of health teaching and health promotion.

Outcomes of actual care practices affect patients and their families, practitioners, and the health care setting. Impacts for patients and their families include obvious health outcomes, their gains in health knowledge, and their satisfaction with care. Care practices affect practitioners' job satisfactions and dissatisfactions as well as their professional self-images. Finally, the way in which care is delivered affects the setting itself, both in its structure and activities and its costs and revenues. All these changes in turn change the health care setting.

Methods for Evaluating Changes

Designing research to document the impacts of an innovation on the health care setting is difficult, because neither the adopters nor the researcher can fully predict what changes may occur. What frequently happens is that only the intended impacts, such as changes in health outcomes or lower costs, get examined systematically. A second challenge is that the wide array of possible impacts means multiple questions requiring multiple methods of inquiry. Philosophically, one could argue that qualitative strategies are more compatible with a research question focused on a process of change, as they provide much richer information, with greater sensitivity to the complexity of particular settings. They also provide a way to see the impact of an innovation from the perspectives of those being affected by it, but quantitative methods are generally locked into the perspective of the researchers. (See Delvecchio, 1992; Jenkins, 1992 for overviews of these philosophical issues related to the primary health care setting.) Qualitative studies are highly labor intensive, however, and a project would seldom have the personnel, time, or financial resources to conduct an intensive qualitative investigation of all of these factors. Where feasible, quantitative indicators of structural or attitudinal change may provide limited but important information at a much lower cost. Adding quantitative data can also enhance the representativeness of an essentially qualitative study. The recent discussions of triangulation of methods are helpful in identifying the strengths and weaknesses of specific methods (Knafl & Breitmayer, 1991; Morse, 1991; Wilson & Hutchinson, 1991), although what we propose here is not strictly triangulation. Rather than measuring the same phenomenon by different methods, we are proposing the use of different methods to assess different parts of a health care setting.

In most studies of the impact of an innovation on a health care setting, the researcher will have to identify the key factors most important to the research question and then select the appropriate research methods. Many compromises will be needed to maximize the quality and completeness of the study within the finite time and money resources available.

Table 9.1 summarizes key advantages and disadvantages of commonly used qualitative and quantitative data collection methods. It is important to note that many methods might be better conceptualized as a continuum from qualitative to quantitative. Both interviews and observations can range from completely unstructured, to semistructured, to highly structured lists of questions or checklists of occurrences. There are also two very different types of records: the statistical records already kept by a health care setting and more qualitative records such as notes of meetings.

Table 9.1 Qualitative and Quantitative Methods of Assessing Impacts on Health Care Settings

Method	Used to Study	Advantages	Disadvantages
Qualitative:			
Observation (unstructured, may use video- or audiotape)	Actual practices	Provides "independent" record of behavior Full, "rich" data with context associated	Limited representation of total behaviors High personnel time Difficult to establish reliability
Interviews (in-depth to semi-structured)	Beliefs, values, attitudes of caregivers Culture, health beliefs, and knowledge of clients	Provides insights into the perspective and worldview of those interviewed Full, "rich" data in its context	Limited number of interviews, not wide representation High personnel time Confidentiality especially needed
Records (nonnumeric such as minutes of meetings, decision making)	Health setting's structure, response to innovations	Easily available Low cost Often complete series available	Only reflects "official" view of what should be recorded Not easy to determine bias, what is missing

(Continued)

Table 9.1 (Continued)

Method	Used to Study	Advantages	Disadvantages
Quantitative			
Surveys (usually from other studies)	Caregiver job satisfaction, attitudes, values	Large, representative samples fairly easy to get	Limited, "thin" data
	Client knowledge, satisfaction	Can often compare to other studies	Perspective of the researcher, not the participants
Structured Observation	Actual practices	Easier to focus on behaviors of interest	Perspective of the researcher
		May enable more observations	Less "rich" data collected
		May be able to compare with other settings more easily	Still fairly high cost
Records (Statistics)	Provider, client demographics	Large, representative sample	Limited variety of information
	Organizational characteristics	Low cost	"Thin" data
			Only reflects "official" view of what should be recorded.

The different factors of the health care setting discussed above can each be assessed by one or more of the methods identified in Table 9.1. Many aspects of the context of a health setting can often be assessed using "historical" statistical records kept by the health care setting. Basic information about the number and types of health care providers, their educational background, age, and years of experience in the current and prior settings is often available from personnel records. If a more intimate understanding of providers is needed, such as their values, local or cosmopolitan orientation, and experiences, a more intensive data collection strategy such as in-depth interviews, semistructured interviews, or questionnaires can be used.

Many characteristics of the health care setting can also be gleaned from records, including size, organizational structure, and patient mix (MacLachlan & Hennen, 1992). Interviews with informants in key positions are likely to be the best way to find out a great deal about a particular health care setting and the larger health system within which it operates. Greer (1984) used interviews to examine the power relationship between physicians and hospital administrators and its impact on the types of innovations adopted. Demographic descriptions of the population served are often available from hospital statistics at an aggregate level. Information about the specific health beliefs, knowledge, and cultural values usually requires intensive qualitative data collection (Brody, 1987; Helman, 1991). Even a short questionnaire, however, can provide useful insights into patients' health knowledge, as in Boyle's (1970) documentation of doctors' and patients' very different definitions of common medical terms. An intensive investigation is warranted for a specific cultural group about which little is known or when an innovation may be more acceptable to some groups of patients than others.

Information about actual care practices is more difficult to obtain from existing records. Many health care settings have fairly detailed written protocols about standard procedures for various situations, and these can be a useful source of information. The prevailing philosophy of care and the many environmental constraints on practice, however, are rarely described in written documents. Equally important, what is actually done rarely corresponds closely with written protocols, simply because a protocol captures such a small part of the totality of provider-patient interaction. This is the area where researchers will normally want to invest their energies in more intensive qualitative study. Both observation of actual caregiver-patient interactions and interviews of individuals and/or groups are good strategies for assessing these complex aspects of the health care setting before and after the introduction of an innovation (Crabtree & Miller, 1992; Miller & Crabtree, 1992). Both audiotapes and videotapes have been used for intensive analysis of patient-provider interaction during care (Byrne & Long, 1976; Pietroni, 1976). Strategies such as focus group interviews are especially good ways to elicit prevailing philosophies and other group norms (Krueger, 1988; Morgan, 1992).

The outcomes of health care practices both before and after the introduction of an innovation are of course the area where the greatest amount of work has already been done. This means that many aspects of these outcomes, especially patient health outcomes and setting costs and procedures, are already routinely documented. Both questionnaires and more intensive interviews can be used to look at patients' satisfaction with care and changes in their health knowledge and practices. The same strategies can also be used to look at the job satisfaction and professional self-image of the health care providers. (See Wilkin, 1992 and Frank, 1992 for descriptions of existing questionnaires and scales for assessment in primary health care settings.)

Studying the process of change in a health care setting when an innovation is introduced is likely to be an especially invasive inquiry, raising special concerns about confidentiality. The usual concerns about confidentiality for individual caregivers are heightened, because the relatively few caregivers in a setting make it much more likely that colleagues will be able to identify each other's remarks even when names and other identifiers have been removed. A good way to handle this is to have individuals read and approve quotations from interviews or descriptions from observations before using them in presentations or publications. The researcher also has an obligation to the organization to present information in a balanced way that does not do serious damage to the organization. It is very difficult to keep an organization from being identified, especially in the local area where confidentiality is most relevant. Findings that may reflect negatively on an organization should be discussed prior to their release, so that the organization can prepare its response (see Chapter 10 in this volume for a more detailed discussion of these issues).

Studying health care settings also raises issues of access. When the caregivers themselves and the setting are being studied, the level of cooperation needed is much higher than when only patients and patient outcomes are looked at. There is often considerable suspicion about the researcher's trustworthiness regarding confidentiality and use of information in a way that does not damage the participating professionals and setting. Qualitative studies often require long and intense data collection that demands time and invades the privacy of workers. A frank discussion of the benefits of the study, confidentiality needs and how they will be assured, and a realistic estimate of the time and level of cooperation needed will help the health care setting make an informed decision to participate.

This discussion of research strategies has been highly abstract. An example of a current project that explicitly studied aspects of a health care setting that may be influenced by an innovation may help to illuminate the complex practical and ethical issues involved in this type of research.

An Example: Describing a Labor Unit

This example is an attempt to study systematically the factors in the labor and delivery unit of a university hospital that affect the way labor is managed prior to introducing a change in care practices (Norr & Roberts, n.d.; Roberts, Norr, & Tunney, n.d.). We have tried to collect at least some information about all of the factors identified above, focusing mainly on actual work practices and the prevailing philosophy of care.

CURRENT CARE PRACTICES

To document current care practices, we used semistructured observations of caregiver behaviors during 60 labors. We had developed a set of key behaviors, verbal statements, and events of interest in a previous study using videotapes. Focused group interviews and questionnaires with doctors, nurses, and midwives were used to develop an understanding of the overall management philosophy and variations in that philosophy by type of practitioner. Environmental factors, including the physical setting and work load, were both observed and asked about during the focused group interviews (Roberts et al., n.d.). Existing records were used about the number and type of care providers and the demographics of the population served. Patient outcomes from medical records were also linked with our observations. We have not yet attempted to assess satisfaction of patients and their families or of the practitioners.

GAINING ACCESS

In this study we encountered different issues of access for the observations of labor and the focus groups with care providers. We began the study with broad general support from the hospital administration and the head of the department and other persons in key positions of authority. In order to conduct our research, however, it was essential to gain the trust and active cooperation of the actual providers.

Being observed with patients can provoke considerable anxiety on the part of caregivers, especially in a setting where many of them are in training and not yet fully confident of their own skills. One barrier is the concern that the information will be used to evaluate individual professional abilities. A related concern in our litigious society is that the observer may witness some critical error on the part of a provider. We used a number of strategies to ease these concerns. We presented the study at formal meetings of the residents, midwives, and nurses. We posted a description of the study in the unit and discussed what we were doing with the resident and nurse in charge each time we came for observation. We then asked them to identify suitable patients and to ask the caregiver to participate. This made it easier for the caregiver to decline. If the caregiver gave preliminary agreement, we then talked about the study to the midwife or resident and the primary nurse for that patient. One reassurance that was very helpful was the reminder that we would leave at any time the caregiver or the patient requested. We approached patients to ask them to partici- pate only after the caregivers indicated willingness to be observed. At first we had a fair number of refusals from care providers, but as we were around the unit more people gradually became more comfortable and the refusal rate declined. In this setting, we had very few refusals from patients throughout the study. Nevertheless, because the study site was large, with numerous caregivers working often irregular schedules, we occasionally encountered people who had not been introduced to the study and had to repeat our time-consuming introduction.

The issue for the focus groups was not apprehension but reluctance to take the time out of a busy schedule to come. Here, personal letters of introduction, careful scheduling of times for staff convenience, inclusion of food at meetings, and follow-up reminder phone calls were all helpful. Caregivers did not seem concerned about confidentiality for the focus group discussions, because as they were talking in front of their peers what they said was already semipublic within this group. Confidentiality and trust may, however, be more problematic for focus groups in other settings or on different topics.

These access concerns raise the interesting question of whether research about health care settings is easier to conduct for insiders or outsiders. Insiders may have an easier time getting initial access from those in authority because they will be trusted more to consider the good of the organization in using and publishing their information. Workers actually participating in the study, however, may be more concerned about possible performance evaluation and about maintaining their professional image with a known colleague than with a stranger.

COMPARING PHILOSOPHY OF CARE AND ACTUAL PRACTICES

At this setting, the two types of caregivers who managed labor— the obstetric residents and the nurse-midwives—had clear differences in their philosophies of care that were identified in the focus groups. The residents had a high-risk orientation to care, and they also revealed that much of their management strategy was dictated by what they felt was an overwhelming environmental pressure of an overcrowded facility. Their basic strategy was to get their patients delivered as quickly as possible, using pitocin for induction and labor augmentation liberally and giving nearly all patients epidurals. The nurse-midwives had a philosophy of non-intervention, but found that they too used interventions more frequently than they might in another setting. These philosophical differences corresponded to differences in caregiving practices, even though we observed only low-risk patients who could have been cared for by either residents or nurse-midwives. Nurse-midwifery patients had lower use of epidural, pitocin, and episiotomy, and longer second-stage labors. The complementary use of two different qualitative techniques, observation and focus groups, supplemented by quantitative information from existing records, provided a rich description of the context of care in a particular setting that could not have been obtained from any single method.

Implications

Research into the impact innovations have on health care settings can make important theoretical and practical contributions. Understanding the difficulties that health care settings encounter can lead to more systematic and reality-based strategies for overcoming obstacles and for identifying interventions that are feasible for widespread adoption. The practical difficulties of studying the impacts of innovations are many, however. Researchers have limited time and resources, and they must set priorities and invest their time and energy where they anticipate the greatest impact of the innovation will occur. Confidentiality and access to the health care setting are important issues, and researchers need to be sensitive to the politics of the setting and the feelings and concerns of participants. This is a research area where much can be gained by linking qualitative and quantitative strategies. Understanding the range of possible methods, their strengths and weaknesses, and the questions each can address will help researchers design methodologically strong and feasible studies of the impacts of an innovation.

References

Boyle, C. M. (1970). Differences between patients' and doctors' interpretation of some common medical terms. *British Medical Journal, 2,* 286-289.
Brody, H. (1987). *Stories of sickness.* New Haven, CT: Yale University Press.

Byrne, P. S., & Long, B. E. L. (1976). *Doctors talking to patients*. London: HMSO.

Crabtree, B. F., & Miller, W. L. (1992). The analysis of narratives from a long interview. In M. Stewart, F. Tudiver, M. J. Bass, E. V. Dunn, & P. G. Norton (Eds.), *Tools for primary care research* (pp. 209-220). Newbury Park, CA: Sage.

Delvecchio, M. J. (1992). Good qualitative designs for assessing intervention. In M. Stewart, F. Tudiver, M. J. Bass, E. V. Dunn, P. G. Norton (Eds.), *Tools for primary care research* (pp. 96-105). Newbury Park, CA: Sage.

Frank, S. H. (1992). Appendix: Inventory of psychosocial measurement instruments useful in primary care. In M. Stewart, F. Tudiver, M. J. Bass, E. V. Dunn, & P. G. Norton (Eds.), *Tools for primary care research* (pp. 229-270). Newbury Park, CA: Sage.

Greer, A. L. (1984). Medical technology and professional dominance theory. *Social Science and Medicine, 18*(10), 809-817.

Helman, C. G. (1984). The role of context in primary care. *Journal of the Royal College of General Practitioners, 34*, 547-550.

Helman, C. G. (1991). Research in primary care: The qualitative approach. In P. G. Norton, M. Stewart, F. Tudiver, M. J. Bass, & E. V. Dunn (Eds.), *Traditional and innovative approaches* (pp. 105-121). Newbury Park, CA: Sage.

Jenkins, J. H. (1992). Theoretical considerations of qualitative method: Behavioral science research of relevance to primary care intervention. In F. Tudiver, M. J. Bass, E. V. Dunn, P. G. Norton, & M. Stewart (Eds.), *Assessing interventions: Traditional and innovative methods* (pp. 69-79). Newbury Park, CA: Sage.

Knafl, K., & Breitmayer, B. (1991). Triangulation in qualitative research: A conceptual clarity and purpose. In J. Morse (Ed.), *Qualitative nursing research: A contemporary dialogue* (pp. 226-239). Newbury Park, CA: Sage.

Krueger, R. A. (1988). *Focus groups: A practical guide for applied research*. Newbury Park, CA: Sage.

MacLachlan, R. A., & Hennen, B. (1992). The medical record as a source for information for research. In M. Stewart, F. Tudiver, M. J. Bass, E. V. Dunn, & P. G. Norton (Eds.), *Tools for primary care research* (pp. 169-176). Newbury Park, CA: Sage.

Miller, W. L., & Crabtree, B. F. (1992). Depth interviewing: The long interview approach. In M. Stewart, F. Tudiver, M. J. Bass, E. V. Dunn, & P. G. Norton (Eds.), *Tools for primary care research* (pp. 194-208). Newbury Park, CA: Sage.

Morgan, D. L. (1992). Designing focus group research. In M. Stewart, F. Tudiver, M. J. Bass, E. V. Dunn, & P. G. Norton (Eds.), *Tools for primary care research* (pp. 177-193). Newbury Park, CA: Sage.

Morse, J. (1991). Approaches to qualitative-quantitative methodological triangulation. *Nursing Research, 40*, 120-123.

Norr, K. L., Roberts, J., & Freese, U. (1989). The impact of rooming-in on maternal attachment. *Journal of Nurse-Midwifery, 34*, 85-91.

Norr, K. L., & Roberts, J. (n.d.). *Care philosophies and patient management styles of nurse-midwives and obstetric residents*. Manuscript under review.

Pietroni, P. (1976). Non-verbal communication in the general-practice surgery. In B. Tanner (Ed.), *Language and communication in general practice* (pp. 162-179). London: Hodder & Stoughton.

Roberts, J., Norr, K., & Tunney, A. (n.d.). *Care practices in a labor and delivery unit*. Manuscript under review.

Rogers, E. M. (1983). *Diffusion of innovations*. New York: Free Press.

Spiegal, N., Murphy, E., Kinmonth, A. L., Ross, F., Bain, J., & Coates, R. (1992). Managing change in general practice: A step by step guide. *British Medical Journal, 304,* 231-234.

Wilkin, D. (1992). Selecting an instrument to measure the outcomes of health care. In M. Stewart, F. Tudiver, M. J. Bass, E. V. Dunn, & P. G. Norton (Eds.), *Tools for primary care research* (pp. 50-63). Newbury Park, CA: Sage.

Wilson, H. S., & Hutchinson, S. A. (1991). Triangulation and qualitative methods: Heideggarian hermeneutics and grounded theory. *Qualitative Health Research, 1,* 263-276.

10 Dissemination of Research Results Prior to Peer-Reviewed Publication

CAROL P. HERBERT

The dissemination of research results to subjects and participants prior to peer review poses a number of questions. Who "owns" the data, and who is responsible for the results and conclusions drawn from them? Are there principles that should govern early release of data and/or results? What about release of data where interpretation by the researchers is in conflict with that of the individuals and communities on which the research was carried out, or where the results reflect badly on the participants or their community? If results are to be disseminated prior to publication in a peer-reviewed journal, by which means should this be done? Should there be a forum that allows for discussion and feedback to the researchers? Can discussion of the data in the course of a research project legitimately form part of the research process? What if the results released turn out later to be invalid after peer review? Is peer review as value-free as we ascribe it to be?

For each of these questions, there are a number of interested parties who may have different viewpoints and perspectives. A challenge exists to bridge the "three solitudes" of the community, community-based health care researchers, and university-based researchers. For example, the Vancouver-based university researcher who studies and describes alcoholism in a First Nations community in Northern British Columbia may have neither knowledge nor understanding of the anger and frustration of native communities when they read yet another prevalence study that neglects the social context of poverty and cultural breakdown after contact with Europeans.

Who "Owns" the Data and Takes Responsibility for the Results?

Research is seen as a "pure" activity, where data are clean and interpretations are driven entirely by the scientific analysis of the results. There are, however, situations that are less clear. For example, when pharmaceutical companies fund research on particular products, who owns the data? When communities or companies pay for data collection and analysis, have they a right to edit the data that supersedes the right of the investigator to publish the findings?

Historically, a distinction has existed between contract funding and grant funding. The former is provided with the understanding that a "deliverable" will be produced for the contractor at the completion of the project. For example, some research that has relied on data from government ministries has required that publication be approved by ministry staff. In contrast, grant funding requires no approval of the outcome or product, so long as both ethical standards and the principles of science are followed. The informed-consent process by research participants is seen as safeguarding the rights and privacy of individuals. An element of the consent process is the subject's agreement that data belong to the researcher and that publication of data and results is an independent action of the researcher. Most researchers would hold that it is essential to the scientific process that data not be altered or edited by any agent, in particular by a "vested interest" such as the funder. This should hold equally true whether the contractor of the research is industry or a community. In research carried out in self-contained or identifiable communities, however, an element of the consent process may indeed be the opposite premise: that is, that data in fact belongs to the community and that agreement by designated community leaders is required prior to publication of results and conclusions. Examples of such agreements may be found in First Nations communities that have had previous experience with outside researchers who have drawn conclusions that have embarrassed the community, for example, prevalence studies of alcoholism, suicide, or HIV infection. The ownership of the data then depends upon agreement among the interested parties, prior to data collection. In the absence of such agreement, the convention of the research community is that the researcher owns the data.

Careful distinction between what are "data" and what are "interpretations" or "conclusions" drawn from data may assist in negotiation between researchers and research participants as to ownership and rights to publication. It can be argued that participants have a right to raw data, but that the conclusions drawn are the opinions—and therefore the responsibility—of the researcher alone. A conscientious researcher, whether university-based or community-based, will ensure that prior to any research project there is a clear understanding both as to how data will be made available to the participants and their community, and whether conclusions drawn will be discussed prior to release to the scientific community.

I believe that the community-based practitioner who provides access to patients for research feels a particular ethical obligation to patients. A question may be raised as to the ethics of the creation of a patient database for practitioner network research. How must patient consent be obtained for such activity? What about data collected routinely, such as immunization or demographic data: Is there a need for consent for release of such information? I suggest that where data cannot be linked to individual patients or to identifiable subgroups or communities, consent is not at issue. The protection of access to any linked data becomes critical.

What about access to patient data by residents or students? Again, the community-based physician is rightly concerned about the increasing number of projects that involve review of charts or other patient data by learners. It is essential that students and residents clearly understand the ethical implications and obligations of research.

When Should Results Be Released?

It would be useful if we could develop principles to govern how and when results should be released prior to peer-reviewed publication. Such principles must include the following:

- *Whenever unexpected findings from the data suggest that research participants require protection from an intervention, or conversely, that control subjects require access to an active intervention, release prior to peer-reviewed publication may be considered.*

An example of early truncation of a study is the Physicians' Health Study (Steering Committee of the Physicians' Health Study Research Group, 1988), a primary prevention trial among 20,000 U.S. male physicians 40 to 84 years of age. Two treatments were compared with placebo: buffered aspirin (325 mg every other day) to assess its impact on cardiovascular mortality, and betacarotene (50 mg every other day) to assess any reduction in the incidence of cancer.

The trial's aspirin component was terminated after about 5 years, 3 years earlier than scheduled, because the rate of myocardial infarction was already reduced by nearly half among the subjects assigned to take aspirin, although the numbers of cardiovascular deaths were not different. The study organizers felt ethically bound to stop the trial so that control subjects could obtain treatment. In this case, publication of the "preliminary findings" did occur in a major medical publication, the *New England Journal of Medicine*.

- *Release of results prior to publication should be accompanied by a disclaimer in case of later invalidation of the results by the review process and/or additional data.* The Physicians' Health Study is again a good example in that the final report showed that an early trend seen in the frequency of moderate-to-severe or fatal hemorrhagic stroke was no longer statistically significant. Most important, the significant 44% reduction in the risk of myocardial infarction was apparent only in patients over age 50, independently of the baseline risk of coronary disease.

- *A process must exist for revision of information provided to the public if results are later invalidated.* In the case of the Physicians' Health Study, more press was given to the initial findings than to the critical review that appeared 18 months later in conjunction with the final report (Steering Committee of the Physicians' Health Study Research Group, 1989). It seems reasonable to hold the researcher responsible for informing research participants if results are later found to be invalid.

- *The Ingelfinger rule* (Relman, 1981), *which prohibits release to the media prior to publication and requires publication in a single journal, must be respected.*

- *It must be recognized that the research process is not value-free.* How questions are framed and how data are displayed may be affected by the values of the researcher and/or the contractor of research, let alone how results are displayed and interpreted. Release of data and results prior to publication may be particularly advisable when topics are value-laden and differential interpretation may occur, for example, sexual abuse or substance abuse research. A counterargument can be advanced, however, that value-laden research cannot and should not be debated outside of the peer-review arena.

- *Release prior to peer-reviewed publication should continue to be conventional practice within the scientific community, for example, by means of working papers and research symposia.* There is an assumption that a medical audience is capable of both interpreting data and understanding the limitations of early release. It must be noted, however, that while researchers are encouraged to utilize scientific meetings for exchange of results and discouraged from release in the public media, we are less clear about the role of the medical press.

What About Conflicting Interpretations or Data That Reflect Negatively on the Research Subjects?

Data may be interpreted differently by interested parties such as the patient, the patient's parents, the patient's physician, the reader of the report, and the funder. In particular, communities or agencies may insist on the right to veto the release of research findings, if release is seen as possibly jeopardizing the community politically (e.g., First Nations communities may perceive that land claims may be adversely affected by descriptions of the social ills of a particular group).

This potential conflict between the freedom of the researcher and the rights of the community may be avoided by written agreement prior to data collection that all published material will be coauthored and/or that some key persons must agree to publication. Such agreement can allow for the inclusion of alternate explanations of the data, informed by community leaders and/or research participants. An example of such an agreement is the

Haida Gwaii Diabetes Education Project, a collaborative study carried out by the University of British Columbia Department of Family Practice with the community physicians and Haida people in two communities in the Queen Charlotte Islands. This project built upon earlier work on Pap smear screening (Calam, Bass, & Deagle, 1992). Diabetes is highly prevalent in North American natives, affecting as many as 50% of those over 35 among the Pima Indians of Arizona (Knowler, Pettitt, Savage, & Bennett, 1981) and 12% of 45- to 64-year-olds in the Mohawk community of Kahnawake, Quebec (Montour & Macauley, 1985). The aims of the Haida Gwaii project include diabetes prevention before and after diagnosis, change in diabetic education and care, development of diabetic materials that incorporate Haida culture, a better understanding of Haida beliefs about diabetes, and a generic model for preventive health among native people.

In order to achieve these goals, the project was designed as participatory action research, utilizing focus groups of diabetics, family members, elders, and community leaders as the "experts" to talk about Haida attitudes and beliefs about diabetes and lifestyle change.

Groups were facilitated by community health representatives, observed by a university collaborator, and taped and transcribed for later analysis. Understanding the themes generated by the focus groups will allow the research team to develop educational interventions for individuals and community that make sense to the participants, who will be consulted repeatedly in the process. This contrasts markedly with the usual imposition of educational interventions on individuals with diabetes or cardiovascular disease (e.g., exercise programs or weight loss counseling). In this project, research is seen as a community-based activity with accountability to the participants, rather than an exploitation of "subjects" by researchers "from away." The research team includes Haida community health reps, family physicians from the community, university-based family practice faculty (a family physician and a social worker with expertise in qualitative analysis), and consultants in nutrition and anthropology. The research process is participatory and egalitarian, with mutual respect and support of team members.

The team developed working principles that govern the project and revisit these at group meetings. Principles include clear definition of roles and responsibilities, shared recognition, and acknowledgment of contributions of all team members as well as of research participants and community leaders. One of the terms of agreement from the outset of the project is that the Haida community health representatives will coauthor all publications and will liaise with the Band Council.

As part of the research process and in response to the wishes expressed by participants, a community forum will be held to discuss the same questions that the focus groups discussed, as well as possible interventions on a community-wide basis. Another approach to ensure that the community is participant rather than passive was the celebration of a feast in each village at the beginning of the project with traditional foods served that were nutritionally appropriate for the diabetics, speeches and presentations, and opportunity for discussion of the project. Another feast is planned at the conclusion of the project when the results are returned to the community.

Another example of such an agreement was concluded between the University of British Columbia's Department of Family Practice and WAVAW, a Vancouver rape crisis group (Women Against Violence Against Women), with respect to a study on sexual assault. In this study, requirements for WAVAW's letter of support for the university-based project included assurance that individual patients' identities would be protected, that patients would not be harmed or embarrassed by publication of results, and that results and discussion would not appear to "blame the victim" as some earlier studies had done. In recognition of this agreement, the final report of the project was made available to WAVAW prior to submission for publication, and note was made in the published report of ethical concerns in violence research (Herbert, Grams, & Berkowitz, 1992).

How Should Results Be Disseminated?

If data or results are to be released prior to peer review, it is usually preferable that this be done by sending letters directly to participants, or by means of focus groups or town meetings with feedback to the researchers of questions, concerns, or opinions. This approach guards against the sensationalizing or overinterpretation of data that may occur in the media. On the positive side, however, a press release ensures wide dissemination of data.

Conventional reporting includes the development of monographs or reports that are available on demand by participants and other interested parties, whether or not peer-reviewed publication occurs. As indicated earlier, increased preparation and dissemination of working papers would allow for wider access to and discussion of results by the scientific community. Such materials can also be made available to research participants.

These more complete collections of data and analysis allow readers to interpret the data and results themselves. Similarly, papers read at scientific meetings are a conventional forum for data exchange prior to peer review. Such reports may of course be picked up by the lay press or the medical press, sometimes before the researchers want a more general dissemination.

What Are the Risks and Benefits of Pre-Peer-Review Dissemination?

I have already alluded to some risks of pre-peer-review dissemination of data and results to subjects, notably sensationalizing, misinterpreting, or overinterpreting results. Conversely, benefit of early release can be feedback to the researchers such that the project is modified to collect data differently or to ask questions more sensitively or more clearly.

The model for feedback to participants and researchers is participatory action research (Barnsley & Ellis, 1992). In the Haida Gwaii Project example, focus group discussion as to causes and possible intervention in diabetes is being used to develop the intervention strategies themselves. The themes extracted from the focus groups have generated additional questions for the next groups.

In the sexual assault study example, early recognition of risk to parts of the study population from some of the research questions resulted in modification of the method (Templeton, 1993).

Ethical Issues in Dissemination of
Results Prior to Peer Review

For the university-based researcher, peer-reviewed publication carries the most cachet in terms of career and consideration of tenure and/or promotion. Pre-peer-review publication of results may jeopardize acceptance, especially by prestigious journals such as the *New England Journal of Medicine,* which adhere firmly to the Ingelfinger rule (Relman, 1981). Researchers must, however, consider their personal need to publish in the context of both the scientific importance of the results and existing agreements with research participants or communities not to release results in certain circumstances.

In the case of community-based researchers—community physicians, for example—no obligation may be felt to the university or to the peer-review process. Tenure or promotion are irrelevant, and allegiance is felt to the individual patients and to their community. Regardless of the researcher's base, of course, agreements about release of results must be honored by the signatories.

Another issue to be considered is whether the peer-review process can be trusted by researchers to eliminate weak research and ensure publication of important results. Some would argue that the process itself is flawed and more of a "sacred cow" than the research community will acknowledge. If peer review is not always trustworthy, then it becomes essential to utilize other avenues of dissemination of results to ensure public access to important findings. The question then becomes, who decides which findings are "important"? The researcher may be seen to have a vested interest or at least not to be objective about the findings.

In general, even with all its limitations, the peer-review process has been useful in improving the quality of published research.

References

Barnsley, J., & Ellis, D. (1992). *Research for change: Participatory action research for community groups* [Brochure]. Women's Research Centre, Vancouver, BC.

Calam, B., Bass, M. J., & Deagle, G. (1992). Pap smear screening rates for native and non-native women on the southern Queen Charlotte Islands. *Canadian Family Physician, 38,* 1103-1109.

Herbert, C. P., Grams, G. D., & Berkowitz, J. (1992). Sexual assault tracking study: Who gets lost to followup? *Canadian Medical Association Journal, 147*(8), 1177-1184.

Knowler, W. C., Pettitt, D. J., Savage, P. J., & Bennett, P. H. (1981). Diabetes incidence in Pima Indians: Contributions of obesity and parental diabetes. *American Journal of Epidemiology, 113*(2), 144-156.

Montour, L. T., & Macauley, A. C. (1985). High prevalence rates of diabetes mellitus and hypertension on a North American Indian reservation. *Canadian Medical Association Journal, 132*, 1110, 1112.

Relman, A. S. (1981). The Ingelfinger rule. *New England Journal of Medicine, 305*(14), 824-826.

Steering Committee of the Physicians' Health Study Research Group. (1988). Preliminary report: Findings from the aspirin component of the ongoing Physicians' Health Study. *New England Journal of Medicine, 318*(4), 262-264.

Steering Committee of the Physicians' Health Study Research Group. (1989). Final report on the aspirin component of the ongoing Physicians' Health Study. *New England Journal of Medicine, 321*(3), 129-135.

Templeton, D. M. (1992). Sexual assault: Effects of the research process on all the participants. *Canadian Family Physician, 39*, 248-254.

PART III

Changing Practitioner Behavior

11 The Dissemination of Information: Optimizing the Effectiveness of Continuing Medical Education

DAVID A. DAVIS

Background: The Literature on CME

Reviewing the continuing medical education (CME) literature is not a new phenomenon. Several major reviews have been published within the past 15 years (Beaudry, 1989; Bertram & Brooks-Bertram, 1977; Haynes, Davis, McKibbon, & Tugwell, 1984; Lloyd & Abrahamson, 1979; McLaughlin & Donaldson, 1991; Stein, 1980). These reviews have provided strong evidence that most CME interventions affect physicians' beliefs about their learning, and that some effect changes in competency (the ability of the physician to perform in the test situation). Less strong, however, is the evidence for changes in actual clinical performance or behavior, and there is only weak evidence of changes in patient or health care outcomes. This chapter focuses on these latter two areas: change in physician performance and in health care outcomes as a result of CME dissemination strategies.

The nature of the sources of the CME literature is eclectic and often unindexed. This prompted the Continuing Health Sciences Education program at McMaster University, Hamilton, Ontario, to develop and maintain a comprehensive collection of the literature, called the Research and Development Resource Base in CME (RDRB/CME) (Annual Report of the Research and Development Resource Base in CME, 1991). Funded in part by the Canadian and

American Medical Associations and the Alliance for CME, the current RDRB/CME contains approximately 2,000 citations relevant to the fields of continuing medical education and dissemination, including all ways by which physician learning and clinical practice may be altered by instructional or persuasive means. Sources used in building the database include computerized searches of Medline, ERIC, and the social sciences literature; manual searches of the nonindexed literature and retrieved articles; and requests of key informants in CME for relevant articles.

Focusing the Literature: Randomized Controlled Trials of CME Interventions

In light of the need to determine rigorously the role of CME in disseminating knowledge on the performance of physicians in practice and on the status of their patients, we created an organized database of the literature. Because of the size of the literature base, articles chosen for review had to meet the following criteria: the CME intervention had to involve randomized controlled trials; to provide a replicable description of an educational activity or program intended to improve physician performance or patient outcomes; to include an assessment of the impact of the intervention in terms of objectively observed health professional performance (behavior) or patient outcomes; to allow for follow-up assessment of outcomes for at least 75% of study participants; to provide sufficient data for analysis; and the participants had to be at least 50% MDs. This review excluded interventions that used sanctions, rewards, or external controls, but it did incorporate maneuvers such as chart reviews with peers, mailed materials, computer-generated information, and other nontraditional forms of communicating information.

Study results were classified into one of three categories. "Positive" studies were those that found a statistically significant difference between a group exposed to the CME intervention and a control group that received no intervention or a less potent one. "Negative" studies were those finding no statistically significant difference between control and study groups, but that possessed sufficient power to rule out a practically important difference. "Inconclusive" studies found no statistically significant or practically important difference, but lacked sufficient power to demonstrate or exclude that such a difference might exist.

Fifty studies met the criteria outlined above. Ninety percent of these examined the practices or patients of internists, general physicians, or family physicians. The remainder were in obstetrics, emergency care, and pediatrics. Twenty-one studies were in hospital out-patient clinics and units, and 16 took place in private practices. Almost a third of the 50 trials included residents or house staff. Finally, 32 trials analyzed physician performance, 7 looked at patient outcomes, and 11 examined both. Nearly half (23) of the studies focused on comprehensive, clinical management of general medical conditions, including investigation, diagnosis, and treatment. Laboratory and radiologic investigations by themselves were the focus of 11 studies, and the remainder were an equal mix of prescribing practices, patient counseling, and prevention activities.

The scope of interventions subsumed by the phrase *continuing medical education* was quite broad: relatively new interventions included chart reviews, computer-generated information, complex role-reinforcing maneuvers such as practice rehearsal in workshops, academic detail visits (visits by trained physician-educators such as pharmacists), opinion leaders, and more traditional strategies such as lectures and printed materials.

Can CME Change Physician Performance?

Of the 16 Randomized Controlled Trials (RCTs) that focused on physician performance in general patient or clinical management, 12 reported statistically significant changes in physician performance (Davis, Thomson, Oxman, & Haynes, 1992). Four employed opinion leaders or "educational influentials" to modify physician behavior; others used well-crafted instructional methods or computer-generated reminders.

Eleven studies assessed the impact of CME interventions on the use or costs of laboratory and/or X ray use. Of this group, 10 demonstrated positive changes by using a variety of intervention measures (Davis et al., 1992). For example, Chassin and McCue (1986), using didactic sessions, printed materials, and feedback, altered the rates of pelvimetry in obstetrics. Similarly, Everett, deBlois, Chang, and Holets (1983) reported that chart review by a faculty supervisor produced positive, statistically significant changes in both costs and frequency of test ordering.

Of six authors who studied the effects of a variety of interventions on physicians' prescribing behaviors, five described positive changes. Meyer, Van Kooten, Marsh, and Prochazka (1991) compared the effects in reducing polypharmacy of a newsletter versus more extensive activities that incorporated an opinion leader, feedback, and chart review: Both were equally effective. Gehlbach et al. (1984) employed feedback mediated by computer to increase generic drug prescribing in a family practice teaching setting. Hershey, Porter, Breslau, and Cohen (1986) also demonstrated that computerized feedback could significantly reduce prescription costs, but in fewer than half of the measured outcomes. A follow-up study by the same author (Hershey, Goldberg, & Cohen, 1988) using computerized feedback and a newsletter had no effect. Avorn and Soumerai (1983) and McConnell et al. (1982) studied the effects of academic detailing in addition to printed material and feedback in lowering the prescribing of targeted drugs. Detailing was effective whereas simple mailed materials were not effective by themselves.

Interventions designed to assist physicians in patient counseling were reported in six studies. Five of these concerned smoking cessation and used complex educational strategies given as didactic presentations, practice-oriented workshops allowing for "rehearsal" of new skills, reminders, printed material, and patient education materials to change physician behavior. In the pediatric literature, Maiman, Becker, Liptak, Nazarian, and Rounds (1988) showed that print material, coupled with didactic and problem-based sessions, could improve pediatricians' compliance-enhancing skills.

All five studies of primary prevention CME interventions displayed significant changes in at least some major outcomes (Davis et al., 1992). Three used computer-generated reminders to physicians to perform certain tasks and found positive changes in most major measures, and two used a combination of didactic presentation, printed materials, and feedback to effect change. The latter two, however, demonstrated significant improvement in only two of eight screening measures in one study, and only in the final 6 months of another.

Although these trials represent a variety of clinical areas, some aspects of clinical practice, such as surgery, were unrepresented. Other aspects—including, for example, data gathering by history and physical examination, diagnosis, procedural or technical skills, the referral process, and information management skills— were rarely studied.

Can CME Change Health Care Outcomes?

Of 18 studies that analyzed the effects of CME interventions on patient or health care outcomes (Davis et al., 1992), including trials in smoking cessation, hypertension, asthma, arthritis, and family practice topics, 10 displayed negative or inconclusive outcomes. There are several explanations for this. First, there may be a lack of direct relationship between the physician performance change induced by the CME intervention and patient outcomes, influenced by the many impediments to optimal outcomes such as patient compliance with medication. Second, a "ceiling effect" may be at work in studies such as those devoted to hypertension, limiting the ability of physicians and patients, already near their maximum capabilities, to improve their performance.

On the other hand, eight of the studies showed a positive patient care outcome in at least one major measure. Two smoking cessation studies (Cohen, Stookey, Katz, Drook, & Smith, 1989; Wilson et al., 1988) demonstrated significant differences in patient quit rates after counseling by trained physicians; Lomas's use of trained opinion leaders increased the proportion of vaginal births after cesarean sections (Lomas et al., 1991); Maiman's mixture of workshop, didactic presentation, and printed materials improved patient compliance (Maiman et al., 1988); and Vinicor et al. (1987) reported that didactic presentations in combination with protocols, reminders, and patient education strategies, improved outcomes in diabetes. Restuccia (1982) determined that feedback reduced inappropriate patient hospital days; and Linn (1980), in an emergency room setting, demonstrated that a combination of protocols, feedback, and traditional teaching methods produced patient changes (although in fewer than a quarter of the measures studied). Rogers, Haring, Wortman, Watson, and Goetz (1982), using computerized medical records, showed positive outcomes in obesity and renal disease.

What Formats Work Best in CME?

The 50 studies used a total of 74 discrete interventions, all of which, by nature of their educational purpose, contained some element of information dissemination. These 74 interventions were classified using a modification of the PRECEDE method described by Green, Kreuter, Deeds, and Partridge (1980). Figure 11.1 presents a more complete description, listing the typology used, the number of interventions assigned to each type, and their outcomes. As seen in the figure, 15 interventions were classified as Type 1 (using predisposing methods only), 12 as Type 2 (employing predisposing methods with practice-enabling strategies), 31 as Type 3 (predisposing methods plus practice reinforcement), and 16 as Type 4 (interventions that used a mixture of all three previous types).

There appears to be a relationship between the intensity of the intervention and the degree to which outcomes were changed. Type 1 interventions (predisposing methods only) generally demonstrated negative or inconclusive results. It would appear that the criticism aimed at this type of intervention, the fare of most traditional CME providers, is substantiated. Only 7 out of 11 studies displayed positive physician performance changes, and none of the six attempts to change health care status did so.

With regard to workshops, conferences, and lectures, those that did not include intra-session practice strategies failed to produce any change in physician performance. In contrast, workshops that provided more opportunity for case discussion, and particularly those that afforded the opportunity to rehearse or consider practice behaviors, were considerably more effective. This finding supports one of the major tenets of the accreditation of CME: that the determination of practice or learning needs is a necessary prerequisite.

With only two exceptions, printed material exerted no demonstrable effect on physician performance if used alone. It may be that printed material acts as a part of the educational "background

TYPE	FEATURES		NUMBER OF STUDIES WITH POSITIVE OUTCOMES	
	PREDISPOSING (DISSEMINATING)	OTHER	PHYSICIAN PERFORMANCE	PATIENT HEALTH CARE
1	✔		7/11	1/6
2	✔	Enabling strategies, facilitating change in practice	9/10	2/6
3	✔	Reinforcing strategies: reminders, feedback	18/26	6/9
4	✔	Both Type 2 & 3 methods, or complex maneuvers, e.g., opinion leaders, chart review	14/14	5/9

Figure 11.1. Categorization of CME Interventions

noise," as one of many impactors on performance, but its utility as an independent agent is questionable.

In this review, small groups failed to demonstrate either performance change or patient outcome change. It is difficult to say whether this apparent lack of effect is due to inadequate potency of the intervention or to unfocused discussion, but we would urge further research in the area, given its increasing use in North American medical schools and the theoretical basis on which the process is based.

The interventions described as "academic detail visits" were classified as Type 1 if only used to disseminate information, but changed to the appropriate type if feedback or patient materials were used. They appear to be effective change agents, worthy of further study both in drug-prescribing trials and in other clinical areas.

In contrast to Type 1 interventions, those that used enabling and/or reinforcing elements were more effective in changing outcomes. Of the 12 Type 2 interventions (enabling or facilitating practice change), 9 of the 10 studies that assessed physician performance change were positive, as was two of six studies that evaluated health care status. There are a wide variety of maneuvers that fill the criteria of Type 2 interventions. Patient education materials were used effectively in three of four interventions, when coupled with academic detail visits, printed materials, or workshops. Information about specific patients, derived from health status questionnaires or interviews, demonstrated positive effects on physician performance in one study, but failed to change patient outcomes in another (Davis et al., 1992). The dissemination of clinical policies or practice guidelines alone had no effect on repeat cesarean section rates (Lomas et al. 1991). More specific practice protocols or clinical flowcharts, however, coupled with printed materials and workshops, changed physician performance in family practice. Finally, computer-generated information used in two studies by Tierney, Hui, and McDonald (1986) and Tierney, Miller, and McDonald (1990) induced physician performance change.

Type 3 methods consisted primarily of feedback, reminders, or a combination of the two, in conjunction with predisposing techniques. They appear effectively to overcome many of the logistical and sociological barriers to implementing optimum physician performance. Feedback produced positive changes in 10 of 14 intervention studies (Davis et al., 1992), either by itself or combined with didactic presentations, workshops, academic detail visits, and/or printed materials. Two studies (Guillion, Tschann, Adamson, & Coates, 1988; Lomas et al., 1991) demonstrated no change in patient outcomes with feedback, and one (Restuccia, 1982) showed improvement using feedback to physicians relating to patient hospital discharges. Reminders were also frequently used, producing consistently positive results in changing physician performance and with mixed results in changing patient outcomes.

Type 4 activities, which used methods from all three categories, constituted the majority of this group: 10 of 16 interventions described (Davis et al., 1992). They produced positive results in all 8 assessments of physician performance, and in 4 of 7 assessments of patient health care outcomes, including smoking cessation and diabetes management studies that used a mixture of workshops, patient education materials, printed materials, and reminders. The effectiveness of opinion leaders or educational influentials in changing behavior and health care outcomes was displayed by Lomas et al. (1991) in a study of vaginal birth following cesarean section practices. In addition, Stross and Bole (1980) and Stross, Hiss, Watts, Davis, and Macdonald (1983) established the performance-altering potential of educational influentials in the management of arthritis and respiratory disease; patient outcomes assessed in only one of these studies were not altered. The use of opinion leaders appears to be a comprehensive maneuver derived from research on the "educational influential" in community hospitals. Finally, chart review, when employed by a faculty member or supervisor, improved physician performance in three studies (Everett et al., 1983; Martin, Wolf, Thibodeau, Dzau, & Braunwald, 1980; Meyer et al., 1991). Chart review, studied by others from the perspective of competency assessment and (under the rubric of chart-stimulated recall) from that of a CME intervention, appears an effective and comprehensive instrument, incorporating elements of information-sharing, reminders of desirable practices, feedback to the physician, and the opportunity for performance-enabling suggestions.

Conclusions: Implications for the Dissemination of Research Findings

Although this review contains numerous implications for dissemination strategies, we recognized difficulties with depending on findings from this source alone. First, a publication bias may be at work here in which negative or inconclusive studies might not be submitted for publication. Second, RCTs are difficult and expensive to perform and usually require volunteer physicians on whom to test interventions: This may limit the generalizability of these findings to physicians who believe themselves to be reasonably competent and are thus willing to have their performance or their patients' health status scrutinized. Third, although these studies eliminated many of the concerns about contamination and cointervention, they frequently lacked qualitative details of potential help in the delineation of physician management patterns, learning processes, or forces for and impediments to change. Fourth, although the studies were generally well designed, methodologic flaws were apparent: For example, some studies did not provide details of their physician populations or blind their assessors to the intervention group. Fifth, although it appears reasonable to assume that all of the "statistically significant" studies found differences that were clinically important, it is not possible to assume that the "inconclusive" studies ruled out a clinically important effect. Although the strength of the inferences that can be made about the relative effectiveness of different CME interventions based on our overview is limited, these inferences may lead to some helpful recommendations for the dissemination of new knowledge.

Despite these cautions, this review reveals the need to address several important issues in the dissemination of research findings by CME methods. First, there are many CME interventions preferred by physicians that have not been studied. For example, journal reading is clearly an important mode of learning about new research findings for most physicians, but it has not been studied to any extent by quantitative methods. Second, there are promising interventions that deserve further testing and use, particularly chart review, opinion leaders, academic detail visits, and staged intervention activities. Third, the clinical outcomes chosen in most CME studies appear to be determined somewhat more by their ease of measurement (e.g., blood pressure) or by their cost (e.g., investigations) than by their clinical imperative. There are several clinical domains, surgery among them, that have not been studied to any extent at all.

Both providers of CME and those entrusted with the dissemination of new knowledge or information need to be aware of the clear lesson derived from this review: that CME is more effective when it incorporates practice-based, enabling, and reinforcing strategies; and that adequate needs assessment leads to increased potential for change. These findings assume importance for the publication and dissemination of research findings or practice guidelines, and call for increased linkages between researchers, CME providers, professional associations, and physicians.

References

Annual Report of the Research and Development Resource Base in CME. (1991). Hamilton, Ontario: McMaster University.

Avorn, J., & Soumerai, S. S. (1983). Improving drug therapy decisions through educational outreach. *New England Journal of Medicine, 308,* 1457-1463.

Beaudry, J. S. (1989). The effectiveness of continuing medical education: A qualitative synthesis. *Journal of Continuing Education of the Health Professions, 9,* 285-307.

Bertram, D. A., & Brooks-Bertram, P. A. (1977). The evaluation of continuing medical education: A literature review. *Health Education Monograph, 5,* 330-362.

Chassin, M. R., & McCue, S. M. (1986). A randomized trial of medical quality assurance. *Journal of the American Medical Association, 256,* 1012-1016.

Cohen, S. J., Stookey, G. K., Katz, B. P., Drook, C. A., & Smith, D. M. (1989). Encouraging primary care physicians to help smokers quit. *Annals of Internal Medicine, 110,* 648-652.

Davis, D. A., Thomson, M. A., Oxman, A. D., & Haynes, R. B. (1992). Evidence for the effectiveness of CME: A review of 50 randomized controlled trials. *Journal of the American Medical Association, 268*(9), 1111-1117.

Everett, G. D., deBlois, S., Chang, P.-F., & Holets, T. (1983). Effect of cost education, cost audits, and faculty chart review on the use of laboratory services. *Archives of Internal Medicine, 143,* 942-944.

Gehlbach, S. H., Wilkinson, W. E., Hammond, W. E., Clapp, N. E., Finn, A. L., Taylor, W. J. & Rodell, M. (1984). Improving drug prescribing in a primary care practice. *Medical Care, 22,* 193-201.

Green, L., Kreuter, M., Deeds, S., & Partridge, K. (1980). *Health education planning: A diagnostic approach.* Palo Alto, CA: Mayfield.

Guillion, D. S., Tschann, J. M., Adamson, T. E., & Coates, T. J. (1988). Management of hypertension in private practices: A randomized controlled trial in continuing medical education. *Journal of Continuing Education of the Health Professions, 2,* 239-255.

Haynes, R. B., Davis, D. A., McKibbon, A., & Tugwell, P. (1984). A critical appraisal of the efficacy of continuing medical education. *Journal of the American Medical Association, 251*(1), 61-64.

Hershey, C. O., Goldberg, H. I., & Cohen, D. I. (1988). The effect of computerized feedback coupled with a newsletter upon outpatient prescribing charges. *Medical Care, 26,* 88-93.

Hershey, C. O., Porter, D. K., Breslau, D., & Cohen, D. I. (1986). Influence of simple computerized feedback on prescription charges in an ambulatory clinic. *Medical Care, 24,* 472-481.

Linn, B. S. (1980). Continuing medical education impact on emergency room burn care. *Journal of the American Medical Association, 244,* 565-570.

Lloyd, J. S., & Abrahamson, S. (1979). Effectiveness of continuing medical education, a review of the evidence. *Evaluation in the Health Professions, 2,* 251-280.

Lomas, J., Enkin, M., Anderson, G. M., Hannah, W. J., Vayda, E., & Singer, J. (1991). Opinion leaders vs audit and feedback to implement practice guidelines. Delivery after previous cesarean section. *Journal of the American Medical Association, 265,* 2202-2207.

Maiman, L. A., Becker, M. H., Liptak, G. S., Nazarian, L. F., & Rounds, K. A. (1988). Improving pediatricians' compliance-enhancing practices: A randomized trial. *American Journal of Diseases of Children, 142,* 773-779.

Martin, K. I., Wolf, M. A., Thibodeau, L. A., Dzau, V., & Braunwald, E. (1980). A trial of two strategies to modify the test-ordering behavior of medical residents. *New England Journal of Medicine, 303,* 1330-1336.

McConnell, T. S., Cushing, A. H., Bankhurst, A. D., Healy, J. L., McIlvenna, P. A., & Skipper, B. J. (1982). Physician behavior modification using claims data: Tetracycline for upper respiratory tract infection. *Western Journal of Medicine, 137,* 448-450.

McLaughlin, P. J., & Donaldson, J. F. (1991). Education of continuing medical education programs: Selected literature, 1984-1988. *Journal of Continuing Education of the Health Professions, 11,* 65-84.

Meyer, T. J., Van Kooten, D., Marsh, S., & Prochazka, A. V. (1991). Reduction of polypharmacy by feedback to clinicians. *Journal of General Internal Medicine, 6,* 133-136.

Restuccia, J. D. (1982). The effect of concurrent feedback in reducing inappropriate hospital utilization. *Medical Care, 20,* 46-62.

Rogers, J. L., Haring, O. M., Wortman, P. M., Watson, R. A., & Goetz, J. P. (1982). Medical information systems: Assessing impact in areas of hypertension, obesity and renal disease. *Medical Care, 20,* 63-74.

Stein, L. S. (1980). The effectiveness of continuing medical education: Eight research reports. *Journal of Medical Education, 56,* 103-110.

Stross, J. K., & Bole, G. G. (1980). Evaluation of a continuing education program in rheumatoid arthritis. *Arthritis and Rheumatism, 23,* 846-849.

Stross, J. K., Hiss, R. G., Watts, C. M., Davis, W. K., & Macdonald, R. (1983). Continuing education in pulmonary disease for primary care physicians. *American Review of Respiratory Diseases, 127,* 739-746.

Tierney, W. M., Hui, S. L., & McDonald, C. J. (1986). Delayed feedback of physician performance versus immediate reminders to perform preventive care: Effects on physician compliance. *Medical Care, 24*(8), 659-666.

Tierney, W. M., Miller, M. E., & McDonald, C. J. (1990). The effect on test ordering of informing physicians of the charges for outpatient diagnostic tests. *New England Journal of Medicine, 322,* 1499-1504.

Vinicor, P., Cohen, S. J., Mazzuca, S. A., Moorman, N., Wheeler, M., Kuebler, T., Swanson, S., Ours, P., Fineberg, S. E., Gordon, E. E., Duckworth, W., Norton, J. A., Fineberg, N. S., & Clark, C. M. J. (1987). DIA-BEDS: A randomized trial of the effects of physician and/or patient education on diabetes patient outcomes. *Journal of Chronic Diseases, 40*(4), 345-356.

Wilson, D. M., Taylor, W., Gilbert, J. R., Best, J. A., Lindsay, E. A., Willms, D. G., & Singer, J. (1988). A randomized trial of a family physician intervention for smoking cessation. *Journal of the American Medical Association, 260*(11), 1570-1574.

12 From Research to Policy to Practice: Closing the Loop in Clinical Policy Development for Primary Care

PAUL A. NUTTING
LARRY A. GREEN

> What we have to deplore is not so much the fact that scientists are specializing, but rather the fact that specialists are generalising.
>
> *Viktor Frankl* (1977, p. 5)

For the foreseeable future, the formal development of clinical policies will be an intermediate and defining step between research and efforts to improve the effectiveness of medical care. Current thinking typically links research, policy, and practice in a linear manner, as shown in Figure 12.1a, and reflects a widespread belief in three critical assumptions. First, it is assumed that practicing physicians are a problem—that they tend to be recalcitrant in following standards of good medical practice and should be the targets of aggressive efforts to achieve compliance. Second, it is believed that medical research can and does produce knowledge that is useful and applicable, and that this knowledge, when summarized in formal clinical policies, will substantially reduce the ambiguity and variation in practice. Third, it is assumed that previous failures of formally developed clinical policies to change physician behavior are the result of ineffective dissemination strategies. Thus the main challenge to bringing physician behavior into conformity with practice policies can be seen as a dissemination problem.

Fallacies in this logic include the assumptions that the process is linear and that it starts with research from outside practice. One could reasonably ask, as in Figure 12.1b, what informs research?— and the answer might bring little comfort to the practicing physician. In general, research questions are defined by researchers and investigated with atypical populations in settings that differ from practice, and the resulting answers are often difficult to translate into clinically useful information. Researchers themselves are the major consumers of research; much medical research has simply not been useful in guiding practice.

Clinical policies, specifically practice guidelines, could be of great value to practicing physicians. Physicians are strongly motivated to do the right thing and actively seek mechanisms that relieve anxiety in the face of the ambiguity and uncertainty that is inherent in medical practice. To be most useful, clinical policies would address clinical issues that are seen by practicing physicians as a problem and by their recommendations and guidance reduce this ambiguity. Ideally, such policies would emerge from an ever-evolving process, depicted simplistically in Figure 12.1c, through which knowledge from practice informs policy and improves practice. The relationships among practice, research, and policy are quite complex, however, and are influenced by multiple and sometimes contradictory forces. These influences are discussed below.

Influences on Clinical Practice

Clinical practice fundamentally derives from the burden of suffering in the community intersecting with legitimate healing and societal concepts of health and disease. Among the many inputs to clinical practice are the physician's training and experience; various regulations; payment and reimbursement structures; the availability of services; wishes and preferences of patients, their caretakers, and parents; tradition and habit; and the medical literature. To the busy practicing physician the medi-

Figure 12.1a

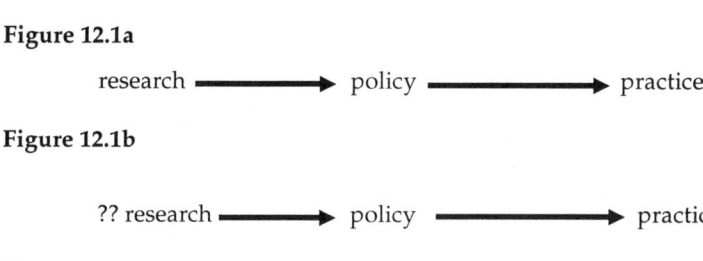

research → policy → practice

Figure 12.1b

?? research → policy → practice

Figure 12.1c

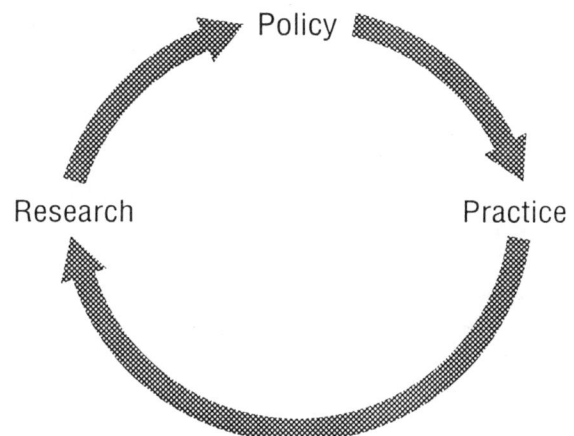

Figure 12.1. The Relationships Among Research, Clinical Policy Development, and Practice

cal literature appears vast, and publication of formally developed clinical policies may bear a striking resemblance to less rigorous review articles by single authors. Especially in primary care, patient factors strongly influence clinical practice. These start with the patient's proposal of a problem in the context of his or her social and economic circumstances, perceived needs, and preferences.

Clinical practice is also strongly influenced by medical traditions. These include the influence of the apprenticeship and the respected authority, the fear of being the first or the last to change, the principle of *primum non nocere,* and the assumption that acts of commission will be forgiven more readily than acts of omission. More recently, practice has become increasingly influenced by certification, recertification, and licensure; the fear of litigation; the effect of public communications media; and practice guidelines from multiple sources.

Patients are perhaps the most powerful determinants of practice patterns. This may be well recognized by physicians as idiosyncracies of certain patients, but is less well recognized as a systematic factor in practice. For example, a parent's expectations of an antibiotic may influence both diagnostic and treatment patterns (Vinson & Lutz, 1993).

Influences on Clinical Policy

Clinical policy derives from the professionalization of healers intersecting with the public's desire to have a check on the mysterious stuff of medicine and healing. Policies are influenced initially by the selection of topics, and major determinants of what is selected include cost of care, mortality, and powerful interest groups including voluntary organizations, payers, and providers. The content of practice policies is influenced by expert opinion, special interest groups, raw political clout, an understanding of uncontrollable variability, the powerful influence of the physician's last/worst/best experience, and research.

Influences on Research

Research is driven by researchable questions from prepared and curious minds intersecting with systems for sustaining researchers. Despite occasional "breakthroughs," research usually proceeds in small increments. Its direction is often determined by the aggregate decisions that researchers make in designing "the next study." These decisions reflect prevailing theory, the researchers' assumptions, and questions identified in previous research. They also depend on access to methods, technology, and clinical phenomena, and to the local infrastructure that supports research.

Last and not least, research depends on the availability of funding, which is largely determined by special interest groups.

The needs of the patients of primary care physicians have not been a powerful determinant of the direction or content of the current medical research enterprise. An emerging exception among U.S. federal research programs is the recently established (but woefully underfunded) Agency for Health Care Policy and Research (AHCPR), which has been given the mission of enhancing the effectiveness of medical practice (Agency for Health Care Policy and Research, 1990).

Reorienting the Effort to Improve Practice

It is possible that difficulties in effectively disseminating clinical policies and changing the practice behavior of physicians is less a failure of dissemination strategies than it is a failure to generate clinical policies that are useful in practice. The improvement of primary care practice will require strategies based on new assumptions. First, we need to recognize the extraordinary opportunities that primary care physicians have to identify clinical problems for which clinical policies can offer a solution. In this way, practicing physicians become a solution rather than a problem. Policies that respond to problems as seen by physicians and their patients, rather than, for example, by third-party payers or governmental agencies, might be more readily adopted by physicians. Second, we must acknowledge that despite its value in advancing basic knowledge of specific disease mechanisms, much medical research to date is not sufficient to address the problems that patients bring to primary care physicians. Third, practice and research can and must be reunited to define and address researchable questions if patients and their physicians are to benefit fully from medical research.

We could reorient our current thinking about clinical policies by changing the starting point in the "research to policy to practice" paradigm (Figure 12.1c). That is, we should let the needs of practice drive the process, and determine: "What is the problem for which this guideline is a solution?"

The Disconnection Between
Primary Care Practice and Research

Even in the United States with its technologically driven health care system, the majority of health care is delivered by primary care physicians (Schappert, 1992). Yet most research is done by others in specialty/tertiary care settings. More than 30 years ago Kerr White and colleagues published a now-classic paper that has changed the way we think about research in primary care, and has provided a new focus for research, based on the relatively unselected patients of everyday practice (White, Williams, & Greenberg, 1961). This paper described the "ecology of medical care" as shown in Figure 12.2a, and quantified the way in which a hypothetical population of 1,000 adults moves into and through our health care system. Of these, approximately three-quarters or 750 individuals will report one or more illnesses or health concerns during a given month. Of these, only one third or 250 people will seek care from their physician. Nine of these will be admitted to a hospital or referred to another physician, and only one will be admitted to a university medical center. Yet most research is done in tertiary care centers where the referral process has concentrated patients who have distinguished themselves in some special way from other patients seen in primary care. Such research is critically important to understanding some aspects of medicine—such as basic pathophysiologic mechanisms that underlie disease and mediate treatments—and it has obvious relevance to the patients selected into the hospital and specialty settings. It does not, however, serve as well to guide primary care practice.

Biomedical research tends to restrict the range of issues under study in several important ways (Task Force on Building Capacity for Research in Primary Care, 1992). First, biomedical research isolates single diseases or disease processes. Much of the research enterprise is designed to understand further the biomolecular mechanisms, diagnoses, and treatments of specific diseases. This often requires that the disease is studied in its fully developed form and in patients without other diseases that would confound the study. In many cases it requires as the focus of study a specific organ, tissue, cell, or intracellular process. Second, disease is studied in highly selected patients. In order to focus on a specific disease mechanism or treatment effect, most medical research

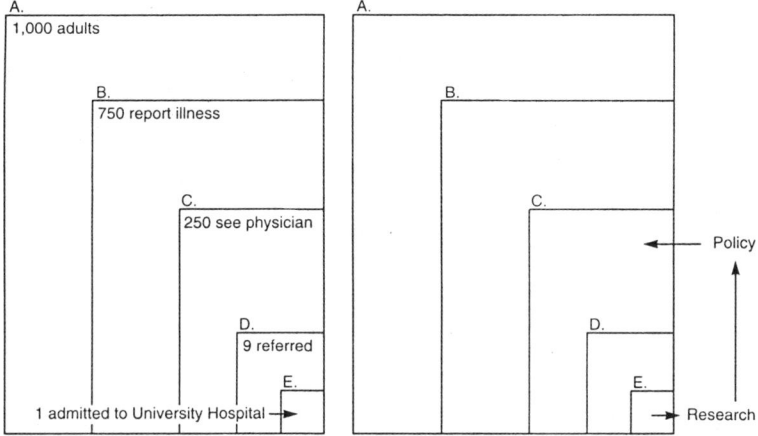

Figure 12.2a   **Figure 12.2b**

Figure 12.2. The Ecology of Medical Care and Its Effect on the Relationships Among Research, Clinical Policy Development, and Practice. In a community of 1,000 adults (Box A), 750 would report an illness during a given month (Box B). Of these, 250 will visit a physician (Box C) and 9 will be referred to another physician or admitted to a community hospital (Box D). Only 1 will be admitted to a tertiary-care hospital (Box E).

carefully restricts the characteristics of the patients under study. Often studies emphasize male adults in their middle years with fully developed disease, without other co-morbidity, and in whom adherence to the protocol can be carefully controlled. Third, most medical research is designed to evaluate single interventions. Although many clinical trials compare several interventions, they are rarely combined in a single arm of the trial in the ways that they are actually used in primary care. Fourth, biomedical research tends to prefer "hard" outcomes, such as death or changes in physical measurements: Less attention is devoted to key personal consequences of effective primary care such as relief of suffering, a sense of having been understood, and the preservation and restoration of function. Finally, the strong focus on disease mechanisms often purposefully excludes the effects of the patients' physical and psychosocial environments, the powerful effects of the physician-patient relationship, and the multiple effects of the system factors inherent in the organization and financing of health care services—all of which are central to the environment of primary care.

Thus much of our medical research has focused on a carefully restricted realm of investigation. Although such research produces critical information for understanding disease mechanisms, it alone is often inadequate to establish practice guidelines that can inform and improve the practice of primary care. Indeed, research in primary care is critical to the development of clinical policies because "it's where so much of the action is." It is where most people go for most of the health problems that bother them most of the time; it is the interface of the health care system with self-care; and it is the interface (through referral) with high-tech, high-cost, and sometimes risky tertiary care.

If we add to the ecology model various influences on practice, research, and clinical policy, a critical disconnection can be seen in relationships among these three elements, as shown in Figure 12.2b. The intended consumers of the clinical policies for primary care (practicing physicians) lack influence on the characteristics of either the policies it is assumed they will value or follow, or the research that is intended to inform these policies. The problems that patients bring to primary care, including many that would benefit from development of clinical policies, can escape detection and careful scrutiny because they are not seen in the settings where most research occurs.

Practice-Based Research Networks

The importance of having a system in place for research is well known. The successes of basic biomedical research have been due to some extent to a network of more than 200 major tertiary care hospitals across Canada and the United States, where specialty care, teaching, and research coalesce in a structure designed to provide access to patients, their diseases, and relevant technology. In contrast, would-be investigators of the relevant phenomena of primary care face substantial logistical problems, as there are no comparable institutions for the less selected populations and ill-defined and relatively undifferentiated problems that present to primary care physicians. One of the most promising developments in primary care research is the emergence of practice-based research networks that have been developed to conduct research on these relatively unselected populations. These networks provide the rudiments of a research infrastructure and provide access to the relevant and somewhat neglected phenomena of primary care, taking its observer and selection biases into account. Critically important characteristics include rigorous attention to research design and in some networks the systematic involvement of practitioners in defining the research questions and participating in the design of the studies. Research questions generated by practitioners and addressed within the practice setting may represent the critical link that connects practice and research. If so, this has important implications for guiding research that will support development of clinical policies.

Practice-based research networks are based on the stronger tradition of research in primary care in Europe and the United Kingdom, and their emergence in North America dates back only a decade. Family medicine has taken the lead in their development in the United States and Canada, manifest by the Ambulatory Sentinel Practice Network (ASPN), the Canadian National Research System (NARES), and several regional networks—notably the Alberta Family Practice Network, the Dartmouth COOP, the Michigan Research Network (MIRNET), and the Wisconsin Research Network (WReN). Research networks have also developed more recently in pediatrics and are under development in general internal medicine.

Informing Clinical Policy Development Through Practice-Based Research

The process of developing clinical policies, that is, practice guidelines, has been carefully defined (Eddy, 1992). Practicing clinicians can participate at virtually every step in the process, but there are at least three critical junctures where their insights and knowledge could be especially important.

The first opportunity is in framing the guideline. This involves not only determining its scope and purpose, but also establishing key assumptions about who will use it, for what patients, at what point, and with what equipment or capacities. The second opportunity concerns the model of evidence to be used in evaluating the guideline. Here, practice-based research can contribute to the identification of the key variables that must be considered, the inclusion of a full spectrum of both potential benefits and adverse effects of the proposed guideline, and assessment of the values that primary care providers and their patients bring to the condition for which the guideline is intended. Third, the practice setting is ideal for evaluating the existence and distribution of key variables involved in guidelines, and for subsequently field-testing their application with special attention to feasibility within the constraints of practice and to the impact that a guideline seems to have on practice.

It takes little imagination to see how practice-based research could improve the chances that a clinical policy framed as a practice guideline would do more good than harm. Through an iterative process, last season's guidelines could be improved and updated. Properly developed, such clinical policies would almost certainly reduce the risk for mistranslation of knowledge from outside the practice setting into practice. Although this process could benefit virtually any guideline, it is critical to those clinical policies aimed at primary care practice, which has distinct needs, opportunities, and barriers that presently are poorly understood. Thus the loop connecting research, policy, and practice could be continuous, reinforcing, and a source of ongoing improvements in practice.

Summary and Conclusion

The desire to improve practice, specifically primary care, is a shared goal of patients, providers, payers, and policy makers. A primary means of accomplishing this is the articulation of state-of-the-art knowledge into guidelines for application in practice, attempting to achieve in practice what works best. The factors that influence research, clinical policy, and clinical practice are sufficiently diverse and complex to make clear why simply organizing what is known and writing it down as a guideline might be neither well received nor implemented. Participation of practicing clinicians during the preparation of guidelines is useful but insufficient when there is a basic lack of understanding of the phenomena of primary care.

If further clinical policy development is to be effective in improving primary care, the primary care physician must be viewed as a solution rather than a problem—as an initiator rather than a passive recipient. To be most effective, development of clinical policies should begin with recognition and definition of specific problems important in clinical practice. Expanded research in primary care settings is essential to inform development of the policies at each of several critical steps—particularly in identifying and framing the topic and in assessing the impact that proposed guidelines are likely to have. Practice-based research networks represent one strategy for uniting practice and research rather than isolating them from each other. Instead of viewing research, policy, and practice in a linear relationship in which practice is understood to be the recipient of important knowledge, the relationship can be conceived as a closed, never-ending loop in which problems from practice inspire research, which informs policy for practice. The nature and perhaps the magnitude of what has been commonly understood to be a dissemination problem would almost certainly change for the better.

References

Agency for Health Care Policy and Research. (1990). *Medical treatment effectiveness research. Agency for Health Care Policy and Research Program Note.* Rockville, MD: Department of Health and Human Services, Public Health Service.

Eddy, D. M. (1992). *A manual for assessing health practices and designing practice policies: The explicit approach.* Philadelphia: American College of Physicians.

Frankl, V. (1977). In E. F. Schumacher *A guide for the perplexed*, p. 5. New York: Harper & Row.

Schappert, S. M. (1992). *National Ambulatory Medical Care Survey: 1990 Summary* (Advance data from vital and health statistics, No. 213). Hyattsville, MD: National Center for Health Statistics.

Task Force on Building Capacity for Research in Primary Care. (1992). *Final report and recommendations of the Task Force on Building Capacity for Research in Primary Care.* Rockville, MD: Agency for Health Care Policy and Research.

Vinson, D. C., & Lutz, L. J. (1993). The effect of parental expectations on treatment of children with a cough. A report from ASPN. *Journal of Family Practice, 37,* 23-27.

White, K. L., Williams, T. F., & Greenberg, B. G. (1961). The ecology of medical care. *New England Journal of Medicine, 265,* 885-892.

13 Integrating Research Findings Into the Clinical Setting Through the Practice of Evidence-Based Family Medicine

TOM ELMSLIE

Ms. Smith sees her family physician because she wants to know if the nicotine patch will help her stop smoking. She is also concerned about the report on a television news program of the deaths of several patients while on the patch. Mr. Jones, who had a vasectomy several years ago, is seen later that day and asks about his risk of prostate cancer and whether he should have the PSA test done, both of which were discussed in a newspaper article. That evening, the family physician reads about the results of a national breast screening study, and wonders how many of the women in her practice are being screened appropriately.

Primary care physicians are required to deal with an increasing amount of medical information about new technologies, interventions, and practice policies found in a variety of sources. These sources include family and general medicine journals, specialty and subspecialty journals and, more recently, the lay press (Phillips, Kanter, Bednarczyk, & Tastad, 1991). Studies that show that effective interventions are slow to make their way into clinical practice may in part reflect the difficulty in trying to keep up to date and synthesizing this information.

Integrating knowledge of the current medical literature into one's clinical practice has not been an easy task, but this is changing. Recent advances in computer technology, coupled with changes in the medical literature, have provided the tools for a new approach called *evidence-based family medicine (EBFM)*. This chapter explores how and whether this approach can be practical and useful.

Evidence-Based Family Medicine

ANSWERING PATIENT-BASED QUESTIONS

The term *evidence-based medicine* has been used by Guyatt (1991) to identify a new approach to medical practice and has been described within the context of the internal medicine specialty (Evidence-Based Medicine Working Group, 1992). This approach emphasizes the use of evidence from the clinical research literature to assist physicians in making clinical decisions about specific patient issues. The four components used in addressing a patient-based question are (a) formulating the question, (b) identifying and retrieving the key article(s), (c) critically appraising this information, and (d) applying the results.

Although the physician must have the skills to carry out effective computerized literature searches and to appraise the articles critically, these skills relate to only two of the four components. The other two components, which start and end this process, are equally important but are often neglected. To start the process, the physician must ask questions that are clinically relevant: for example, areas of treatment, investigations, preventive care, and prognosis. Questions are most often triggered by a specific patient encounter. The way in which the question is posed is crucial in directing the literature search and will ultimately be the key factor in whether the best available information is obtained. The final component requires the physician to be able to apply this information to the unique context and preferences of a specific patient. In family practice there are often no definitive answers and knowing that the evidence does not support one particular choice allows the physician to be more flexible in the decision-making process.

We call the process of using these four components a *patient-based clinical* vignette. The term "critical appraisal" has been purposely avoided in this phrase because we do not wish to emphasize only one part of the process. Although critical appraisal is an important component, it is usually taught in a seminar or work-shop setting; because it is not shown how it can be integrated into the clinical setting, it often remains more of an academic exercise than a clinically useful tool. The clinical vignette format provides one approach that links critical appraisal to clinical decisions about a specific patient.

ANSWERING PRACTICE-BASED QUESTIONS

Unlike the subspecialist, the family physician is interested in continuity of care not only of individuals but also of a practice; and family medicine offers the unique opportunity to expand the scope of inquiry to include questions about one's practice as well as about specific patients. As shown in Figure 13.1, this type of question is more complex and requires additional skills and re-sources. The *practice-based clinical* vignette includes two additional components: (a) computerized access to the appropriate practice information, and (b) comparison criteria based on the best avail-able evidence from the literature. Evidence-based family medicine implies a broader application of the use of evidence than that described by Guyatt (1992) and colleagues for internal medicine.

In a practice-based clinical vignette, the literature search in-cludes review articles, meta-analysis, and various types of practice policy articles. Critical appraisal of these articles provides the comparison criteria with which family physicians can assess their practice information.

The practice-based clinical vignette may appear to be similar to the medical audit loop as described by Shaw (1980) and Derry et al. (1991); however, there are significant differences. In order for the medical audit to achieve the level of scientific rigor required by regulatory bodies and for research studies, it has taken on an external perspective with regards to the family physician. Often it consists of a one-time, general assessment of overall practice quality, with little clinical relevance to individual physicians and uses minimal standards for comparison because the objective is to identify physicians who practice in an unacceptable manner. The physician has a passive role in the process. This external perspec-tive may explain why the medical audit has not gained wide acceptance within primary care as a method for physicians to improve the way they practice.

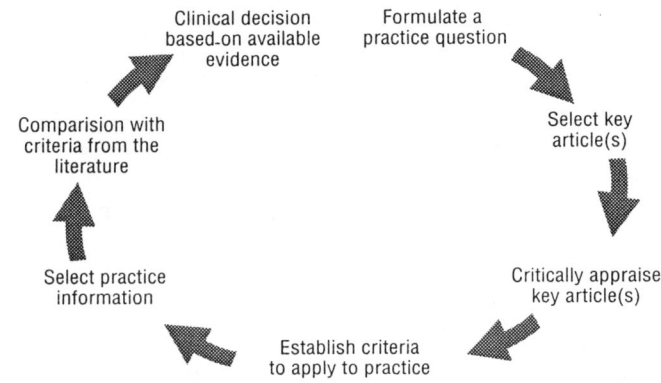

Figure 13.1. Practice-Based Clinical Vignette

The opposite is true of the practice-based clinical vignette of EBFM. Practice questions are formulated that are clinically relevant to the individual physician, and it is the physician him- or herself who assesses the evidence from the literature in identifying the highest level of care with which to compare the practice information. The result will either reinforce the current practice or identify the need for change. Repeating the same question at a later date not only updates the comparison criteria, but provides the physician with a measure of change over time.

Is Evidence-Based Family Medicine Feasible?

Is it possible for busy family physicians to practice EBFM? Until recently, the answer would have been a resounding No! Key changes over the past 5 years, however, in the areas of computerized literature searching, the medical literature itself, critical appraisal strategies, and computer access to patient practice information have opened up new possibilities.

COMPUTERIZED SEARCHING OF THE MEDICAL LITERATURE

The days of physically going to the library, doing a manual search of Index Medicus, and locating the journals are long past. This is equally true of the librarian-directed computerized literature search. Access from one's own office or home to the computerized medical literature is now inexpensive and practical, and the cost of owning a computer, modem, and printer is no longer a prohibitive factor. There are many medical literature databases to which one can subscribe, and the communications software to connect to these databases is now simple to use and once set up requires little attention. The National Library of Medicine's Medline medical literature database is probably the one most commonly used by physicians. Medline can be accessed either directly, using search software such as Grateful Med, or by linking to a CD-ROM/Medline system subscribed to by a nearby hospital or academic center. The CD-ROM/Medline's search software packages, such as CDPlus, usually allow for both menu-driven strategies for the computer novice and more sophisticated approaches for the expert user. (At the University of Ottawa, the Family Medicine department started directly accessing Medline with Grateful MED and, as the number of searches increased, found that it was more cost-effective to use a single user CD-ROM/Medline system. We have recently expanded to a multiuser CD-ROM/Medline system as the demand for literature searching by our faculty and residents continues to increase. All access to our system is by modem from individual office sites, both academic and community based. The easy use of the software has surprised many of the new users, and MESH—Medical Subject Headings—is no longer thought of as a four-letter word.)

Expansion of library services and the use of fax machines have made the retrieval of key articles a convenient process. For those articles needed yesterday, full-text medical databases such as BRS Colleague allow immediate downloading and printing of the complete article. The family physician of the 1990s has easy and inexpensive access to the medical literature.

CHANGES TO THE MEDICAL LITERATURE

Along with improved access to the medical literature, there have been important changes occurring in the literature itself. Structured abstracts for articles of original research are now required by most of the major journals used by family physicians (Haynes, Mulrow, Huth, Altman, & Gardner, 1990). The information in these abstracts allows the reader better to select and retrieve only those articles likely to be useful in addressing a specific patient or practice question. As well, medical editors now require review articles to be more systematic and critical in their assessment of a topic (Squires, 1989). The number of articles using meta-analysis methodology has also increased and provides the reader with information summarized from many related studies (Sacks, Berrier, Reitman, Ancona-Berk, & Chalmers, 1987). More recently, many types of practice policy articles have been published. The process used to develop practice policies has recently come under closer scrutiny, and the quality should continue to improve as the recommendations are reported in a way that allows the reader to assess the level of evidence that supports them (Haines & Feder, 1992). All these changes bring better information in a form that is more useful to the busy practitioner.

CRITICAL APPRAISAL STRATEGIES

Some years ago, the Department of Clinical Epidemiology and Biostatistics at McMaster University published a series of articles on how to read clinical journals (Department of Clinical Epidemiology, McMaster University Health Sciences Centre, 1981a, 1981b, 1981c, 1981d). These articles provided the first practical method for physicians to take an active role in assessing the medical literature; they form the basis of most critical appraisal seminars given today. The College of Family Physicians of Canada has made available individual critical appraisal packages based on this series but from a family medicine perspective (Litt, Mousseau, & Hutchison, 1986). The availability of these strategies provides the opportunity for most physicians to make their own assessments of original research articles, particularly those focused on therapy, diagnosis, and prognosis.

Challenges have been made that review articles should follow a more systematic and scientifically rigorous approach (Huth, 1987; Mulrow, 1987). These challenges have been met by an excellent article (Oxman & Guyatt, 1988) to assist physicians in critically assessing review articles.

With the increased interest in articles about clinical practice guidelines (Fletcher & Fletcher, 1990), strategies are being developed that will help family physicians assess these guidelines in order to differentiate the excellent ones (those based on a systematic review of the evidence in the literature) from the poorly developed ones (Hadorn, McCormick, & Diokno, 1992).

ACCESSING PATIENT AND PRACTICE DATA

Access to practice data has always been difficult. The traditional medical audit provides a good example of how this difficulty has resulted in a passive role for the physician and offers a good contrast with what is available now.

The chart review has been the method most frequently used to access practice data for medical audits; however, there are many limitations to this approach. Chart abstraction is very time consuming and requires standardization in order to ensure reliable information. Often the patient information needed to make valid observations about the practice is either not in the chart or is incomplete. Moreover, charts need to be selected in a manner that provides an unbiased and eligible sample, and this requires some knowledge of sampling strategies. The data abstracted usually must be entered into a data file for analysis. Chart review is costly and usually requires skills and personnel from outside the practice setting.

Fortunately, computerized medical practices are becoming more common. New changes in computer technology provide easy retrieval of all relevant practice data, removing the issues around sampling and chart abstraction. The cost of these sophisticated computer systems continues to decrease. Changes by the provincial health insurance plans, such as Ontario's recently mandated new billing requirements, will likely accelerate the computerization of family practices. Standards for what should be contained in a computerized medical record are being examined, which will help ensure that computerized practice systems contain at least the minimum required patient information.

In many ways, physicians' access to practice data is at a stage similar to where their access to the medical literature was several years ago. In the next few years, though, family physicians should have a wide choice of systems that will permit easy storage, searching, and retrieval of such data, enabling them to play an active role in answering practice-based questions.

CURRENT BARRIERS

The areas of change described above have been essential in enabling the EBFM approach to become practical in the clinical office setting. There are, however, still barriers to be faced.

For some family physicians, the notion of conducting literature searches from their offices and carrying out critical appraisals of articles in order to answer patient questions will seem quite foreign. Certainly, the routine and time pressures required of a busy practice may not seem to lend themselves to the inquiry required in EBFM. Some physicians may feel that they do not have the skills or the time to learn these skills; even such seemingly simple tasks as learning how to link one's computer to a medical literature database can prove challenging to the uninitiated.

One strategy that will enhance the learning of EBFM is for it to become an integral part of family medicine residency programs, with clinical faculty acting as role models and facilitators. This has proved to be a successful approach at our family medicine residency program at the University of Ottawa. Strategies that will enable established practitioners in the community to acquire these skills still need to be developed.

Is Evidence-Based Family Medicine Clinically Useful?

Even if EBFM proves to be practical, several key questions remain to be answered. Will practicing EBFM:

1. change physician behavior?
2. integrate research findings into the practice setting?
3. improve patient health outcomes?

At present, no studies are available that directly provide answers to these questions; however, indirect evidence from the literature and experience at centers such as ours at the University of Ottawa suggest that EBFM is a promising approach. The literature on continuing medical education (Davis, Thomson, Oxman, & Haynes, 1992; Manning & DeBakey, 1992), on the use of the medical audit in England (Mugford, Banfield, & O'Hanlan, 1991), on practice policy (Lomas et al., 1989) and on quality of care (Berwick, 1989; Merry, 1990) provides some evidence on factors that seem to have a positive influence on the first issue: physician behavior. The important factors identified by this literature include an active physician role that is practice-based, clinically relevant, and has a focus on continuous improvement—the same factors that are emphasized in EBFM. EBFM stresses an active role for the physician—it involves the physician assessing and applying the evidence from the medical literature to a specific patient or practice question that he or she feels to be of particular importance. Perhaps most important, EBFM is a continuous process whereby physicians actively attempt to improve the way they practice.

Conclusions

Physicians who practice evidence-based family medicine make clinical decisions about both specific patient and practice questions based on their assessment of the evidence in the medical literature. This approach requires the integration of critical appraisal skills with the ability to search effectively the computerized medical and patient practice databases in the clinical setting. Recent advances have made it possible for family physicians actively and continuously to assess and change aspects of their practice.

References

Berwick, M. D. (1989). Continuous improvement as an ideal in health care. *New England Journal of Medicine, 320*(1), 53-56.

Davis, A. D., Thomson, M. A., Oxman, D. A., & Haynes, R. B. (1992). Evidence for the effectiveness of CME: A review of 50 randomized controlled trials. *Journal of the American Medical Association, 268*(9), 1111-1117.

Department of Clinical Epidemiology, McMaster University Health Sciences Centre. (1981a). How to read clinical journals: I. Why to read and how to start reading them critically. *Canadian Medical Association Journal, 124*, 555-558.

Department of Clinical Epidemiology, McMaster University Health Sciences Centre. (1981b). How to read clinical journals: II. To learn about a diagnostic test. *Canadian Medical Association Journal, 124*, 703-710.

Department of Clinical Epidemiology, McMaster University Health Sciences Centre. (1981c). How to read clinical journals: III. To learn the clinical course and prognosis of disease. *Canadian Medical Association Journal, 124,* 869-872.

Department of Clinical Epidemiology, McMaster University Health Sciences Centre. (1981d). How to read clinical journals: V. To distinguish useful from useless or even harmful therapy. *Canadian Medical Association Journal, 124,* 1156-1162.

Derry, J., Lawrence, M., Griew, K., Anderson, J., Humphreys, J., & Pandher, K. S. (1991). Auditing audits: The method of Oxfordshire Medical Audit advisory group. *British Medical Journal, 303,* 1247-1249.

Evidence-Based Medicine Working Group. (1992). Evidence-based medicine. *Journal of the American Medical Association, 268,* 2420-2425.

Fletcher, H. R., & Fletcher, W. S. (1990). Clinical practice guidelines. *Annals of Internal Medicine, 113,* 645-646.

Guyatt, G. H. (1991). Evidence-based medicine. *Annals of Internal Medicine, 114* (ACP J Club. suppl. 2), 1-16.

Hadorn, D. C., McCormick, K., & Diokno, A. (1992). An annotated algorithm approach to clinical guideline development. *Journal of the American Medical Association, 267,* 3311-3314.

Haines, A., & Feder, G. (1992). Guidance on guidelines. *British Medical Journal, 305,* 785-786.

Haynes, R. B., Mulrow, C. D., Huth, E. J., Altman, D. G., & Gardner, M. J. (1990). More informative abstracts revisited. *Annals of Internal Medicine, 113*(1), 69-76.

Huth, E. J. (1987). Needed: Review articles with more scientific rigor. *Annals of Internal Medicine, 106,* 470-471.

Litt, J. C. B., Mousseau, J. M. D., & Hutchison, B. G. (1986). *Critical appraisal package: Therapy.* Toronto: College of Family Physicians of Canada.

Lomas, J., Anderson, G. M., Dominick-Pierre, K., Vayda, E., Enkin, M. W., & Hannah, W. J. (1989). Do practice guidelines guide practice? The effect of a consensus statement on the practice of physicians. *New England Journal of Medicine, 321*(19), 1306-1311.

Manning, P. R., & DeBakey, L. (1992). Lifelong learning tailored to individual clinical practice. *Journal of the American Medical Association, 268,* 1135-1136,

Merry, D. M. (1990). Total quality management for physicians: Translating the new paradigm. *Quarterly Review Bulletin, 16,* 101-105.

Mugford, M., Banfield, P., & O'Hanlan, M. (1991). Effects of feedback of information on clinical practice. *British Medical Journal, 303,* 398-402.

Mulrow, C. D. (1987). The medical review article: State of the science. *Annals of Internal Medicine, 106,* 485-488.

Oxman, A. D., & Guyatt, G. H. (1988). Guidelines for reading literature reviews. *Canadian Medical Association Journal, 138,* 697-703.

Phillips, D. P., Kanter, E. J., Bednarczyk, B., & Tastad, P. L. (1991). Importance of the lay press in the transmission of medical knowledge to the scientific community. *New England Journal of Medicine, 325,* 1180-1183.

Sacks, H. S., Berrier, J., Reitman, D., Ancona-Berk, V. A., & Chalmers, T. C. (1987) Meta-analysis of randomized controlled trials. *New England Journal of Medicine, 316,* 450-455.

Shaw, D. C. (1980). Aspects of the audit: 4. Acceptability of audit. *British Medical Journal, 280,* 1443-1446.

Squires, B. P. (1989). Biomedical review articles: What editors want from authors and peer reviewers. *Canadian Medical Association Journal, 141,* 195-197.

14 External Support Can Change Primary Care Practice Patterns

ALLEN J. DIETRICH

A current focus of health care research and policy is the development of practice guidelines. How best to support application of such guidelines is open to question, however. Greer (1988) has observed that "there are no magic signatories or formats that will cause knowledge to jump off a page and into practice" (p. 23). This chapter addresses the jump from published guidelines to physician practice, with special attention to the potential impact of facilitators—nonphysician consultants who can assist practices to improve the organization and process of care provided. First, we describe the facilitator model and studies that support its efficacy in promoting the adoption of guidelines in practice. Then, we discuss the stages of adopting guidelines and how to encourage this process through various means that fit the unique needs and characteristics of individual practices.

The Facilitator Model

In the Oxford Prevention of Heart Attack and Stroke Project (OXCHECK), Fullard, Fowler, and Gray (1984, p. 1586) "provide practices with additional energy required to change working patterns. . . . What primary care teams need is not more exhortations,

AUTHOR'S NOTE: This research was supported by grants CA52631, CA54300, CA23108, and F06TWO1643 from the National Cancer Institute, Washington, DC.

or even more knowledge, but practical help to reorient their activity . . . and practise preventive medicine." OXCHECK facilitators assisted practices to:

discuss prevention and set objectives,

train a practice nurse in dietary and smoking cessation counseling as well as in other aspects of prevention,

encourage practice staff to recruit patients in need of these services as opportunities present,

develop tools such as reminder labels and recall systems that support preventive care, and

set up a system of audit to measure progress.

During the past decade, the role of facilitators in Britain has expanded substantially. The National Health Service employs more than 200. Facilitators now address asthma, diabetes, and a broad range of other clinical areas, as well as preventive and general management issues such as team building (Pritchard & Pritchard, 1992) and audit (Gray, O'Dwyer, Fullard, & Fowler, 1987). The typical facilitator has experience in primary care, may be a nurse, is employed by a National Health Service regional office, and works with practice physicians, nurses, and other staff on request. Facilitators do not care for patients in the office, but provide management consultation and assistance with the process of change. Resource workbooks, manuals, and videotapes support them in their work (Roberts, 1991), and the Association of Primary Care Facilitators provides training workshops and other professional development.

The facilitator model may be more familiar to North American physicians than is apparent at first. Large clinical organizations often have an office of quality assurance to monitor and improve the quality and efficiency of care, where nonphysician staff with special training may assist clinicians to assess their performance in the management of target conditions. The clinicians discuss results, identify areas where care can be improved, and then plan and implement the improvements, often with support from these staff. Continuous Quality Improvement (Berwick, 1980) is one such formal approach, with support personnel often functioning in a facilitator role.

The Efficacy of Facilitators in Supporting Change

In a 1987 study, three U.K. general practices that had been provided support by a facilitator reported improved recording of cardiovascular risk factors compared with three control practices (Fullard, Fowler, & Gray, 1987). In the United States, two randomized trials have demonstrated the efficacy of facilitators in modifying physician performance of preventive services: the Doctors Helping Smokers Study (Kottke et al., 1992), and the Cancer Prevention in Community Practice Project (Dietrich et al., 1992)

In the first study, research assistants worked with practice physicians and office staff to help them better assist smokers to quit. As in OXCHECK, these assistants worked as facilitators: training practice nurses to provide counseling; helping office staff take an expanded role in the identification and counseling of smokers; and assisting practices with the implementation of tools such as external chart identifiers, flow sheets to monitor patients' progress, and patient education materials.

The Cancer Prevention in Community Practice Project consisted of a randomized trial of interventions designed to improve physician performance regarding early detection and preventive services as defined by the National Cancer Institute (1987). In New Hampshire and Vermont, 98 family physician and general internist practices received either physician education; assistance from a facilitator in improving those office routines that support age- and gender-appropriate cancer early detection/preventive care; both physician education and facilitator assistance; or neither. Compared with control practices after 12 months, those practices that received facilitator assistance provided significantly more indicated clinical breast examinations and mammograms, and four of eight other target services. Physician education in addition to facilitator assistance provided no incremental improvement. Those practices that received physician education alone provided more mammography than controls, but showed no difference for the other nine target services.

In these two projects, as well as the OXCHECK project described earlier, the successful intervention was based on an expanded role for office staff, use of tools such as chart identifiers and flow sheets, and the development and implementation of a formal office system consisting of defined routines and personnel responsibilities. A hallmark of all these projects was the flexibility of the facilitator's approach in assisting each practice to evaluate current operations and outcomes, modify routines and staff responsibilities, select and customize tools that improve the process of care, encourage quantitative assessment such as audit, and support the change process over time. The facilitator approach differs from many other community practice prevention studies in which research assistants apply a tightly defined intervention such as use of a standard flow sheet or an expanded role for an office nurse. It also differs from many Continuous Quality Improvement efforts (Kritchevsky & Simmons, 1991) in that self-monitoring of performance is encouraged but not required.

Less flexible approaches may apply to practices that eagerly want help, that function with close administrative control (as in managed care), or that include training programs. Openness and ability to change vary between practices and over time within practices; and the physicians and staff of a practice are the ones who understand its needs and resources best. External assistance may be needed to overcome a practice's inertia, to develop its resources, and to help it move from its current performance to the levels of care described in guidelines. This external assistance must, however, come on terms that the practice can accept.

Guidelines as Innovations and the
Readiness of Practices to Adopt Them

Although recognizing that some aspects of any guideline may be familiar to physicians, Kaluzny et al. (1991) consider newly published guidelines to be innovations and have proposed that practices fit various stages in their readiness to adopt them. These stages include:

Recognition that providing guideline services is a legitimate practice function,

Identification that an explicit practice policy and a systematic approach are necessary to provide high-quality care as defined by the guidelines,

Implementation of the systematic approach initially, and
Maintenance or institutionalization of the system.

We draw a distinction between the physician knowledge
necessary to reach the Recognition and Identification stages,
and the practice routines and infrastructure that make the practice environment conducive to ongoing application of the guidelines in the Implementation and Maintenance stages. At the
start of the three projects described here—OXCHECK, Doctors
Helping Smokers, and the Cancer Prevention in Community
Practice—the participating physicians and their staffs already
considered preventive care to be useful, important, and part of
their practices: that is, they had reached the Recognition stage.
All knew about the various indicated services and many had a
policy, albeit usually unwritten and informal, about the services
they intended to provide: Thus they had also reached the Identification stage.

Few, however, had reached the Implementation or Maintenance
stages. In the practices that had, the systematic approach used was
based almost exclusively in the hands of the physicians, who
received little support from their office staffs or from flow sheets
or other organizational aids. Taking advantage of opportunities to
provide preventive care outside of periodic health examinations
was haphazard and uncommon, subject to the distractions and
pressures that are part of clinical practice. For most of these
practices, sufficient knowledge was in place but supportive practice environments were not.

Most guideline dissemination efforts emphasize the knowledge needed to reach the Recognition and Identification stages—
getting physicians' attention and advocating a specific systematic
approach. Few, however, address the routines and infrastructural
office staff support that are usually necessary to *apply* the approach and reach the Implementation and Maintenance stages.
Typically, guidelines are developed; announcements follow through
press releases and publications; then the guidelines are revised
several years later and the cycle is repeated.

Some current dissemination efforts do support reaching the
Implementation and Maintenance stages. The American Academy

of Family Physicians (1987) distributes a kit that includes educational materials, chart identifiers, and other aids to establishing a systematic practice approach to smoking cessation, and the United States Preventive Services Task Force Coordinating Committee is pilot-testing a kit entitled Putting Prevention Into Practice (U.S. Department of Health and Human Services, 1992), which includes flow sheets, patient-held records, and other aids to implementing a systematic approach to providing preventive guidelines recommended by the Task Force (U.S. Preventive Services Task Force [USPSTF], 1989). To date however, neither of these programs has been subjected to a randomized trial. They may provide sufficient support for some practices to implement and maintain the guidelines they address, but they both provide less support than do the three projects described above that follow the facilitator model.

Even for the most receptive practices, there may be a dose-response threshold that must be reached for external help to have an impact (Fowler, Fullard, & Gray, 1992). For example, in Australia facilitators delivered smoking cessation kits to general practices and made personal presentations on their use lasting a mean of just 12.8 minutes (Cockburn et al., 1992). These kits included patient aids to smoking cessation (such as quitting contracts), as well as self-help materials. A second visit to the physician followed 6 weeks later. Over the 4-month study period, more physicians who received such visits indicated that they had seen the kit than those who had received it by mail or courier; however, use of the aids provided within the kits was not increased. In contrast, in the Cancer Prevention in Community Practice Project, three visits of 15 to 60 minutes each were the usual minimum, and six or more visits were not unusual (Carney, Dietrich, Keller, Landgraf, & O'Connor, 1992).

How Far Is the Jump: Current Gaps Between Guidelines and Performance

In considering the appropriate role and effective dose of facilitators in future efforts, it is instructive to consider current gaps between expert guidelines and physician performance, as well as other available methods that may assist in making the jump between them.

Inherent in the creation of guidelines is the notion that current physician performance can and should be improved. Perhaps best studied to date is the gap between expert guidelines and physician recommendations for mammography for women aged 50 years or more. The appropriateness of regular mammography for women aged 50 to 59 years is well established (National Cancer Institute [NCI], 1987; USPSTF, 1989), yet the National Cancer Institute Breast Cancer Screening Consortium (1990) found in 1987-1989 that even though more than 90% of women indicated that they had a regular physician, only 26%-43% in this age group had had a mammogram within the past year. The Cancer Prevention in Community Practice Project showed that with facilitator help, practices increased their annual mammography recommendations to this group from 57% to 78% (Dietrich et al., 1992).

Similar gaps may exist in the application of guidelines that address specific diseases. Ford and colleagues studied the diffusion of management guidelines for breast and lung cancer in 17 community hospital oncology programs and found little evidence of their adoption one year later (Ford, Hunter, Diehr, Frelick, & Yates, 1987). Even among most of the physicians who had themselves participated in the guideline development, few applied them in practice. For example, one prominent program guideline addressed documentation of the clinical stage of breast cancer, but only 28.5% of patient records had this information recorded. The ability to create guidelines currently appears to exceed the ability to apply them.

Of course some gaps may be appropriate. Mant (1992) has observed that facilitators can influence physicians to increase services that are of no proven value as well as those that have been proven. Experts are currently divided on a host of clinical issues such as the role of fecal occult blood testing in the early detection of colon cancer (NCI, 1987; USPSTF, 1989) and the role of anti-inflammatory drugs in the management of asthma (McFadden & Gilbert, 1992; National Heart, Lung, and Blood Institute [NHLBI], 1991). In some cases, practicing physicians may wisely be applying a brake to the dissemination of guidelines that lack sufficient expert support to justify widespread application.

Strategies to Promote Implementation
and Maintenance of Guidelines

Strategies that influence the application of preventive clinical
recommendations in individual practice have been reviewed by
Lomas and Haynes (1988), and strategies that influence physicians
to follow cost-containment guidelines have been reviewed by
Eisenberg (1986). The taxonomies they propose are similar and can
be useful in addressing the application of other guidelines as well.

Professional education strategies such as publication in medical
journals (NHLBI, 1991), word of mouth from influential physicians (Coleman, Katz, & Menzel, 1966), and formal continuing
medical education programs have been the traditional bearer of
practice guidelines as well as most other new clinical information.
Patient-centered strategies include encouraging patients to take
an active role in their care through coaching by non-clinician staff
(Greenfield, Kaplan, Ware, Martin, & Frank, 1988) and providing patient education materials. Administrative strategies include
office reminder systems (McPhee, Bird, Fordham, Rodnick, &
Osborn, 1991), an increased role for office staff (Dietrich et al.,
1992), and feedback to physicians on their performance (Tierney,
Hui, & McDonald, 1986). Economic strategies include incentives
for guideline compliance (Chomet & Chomet, 1990). Lomas and
Haynes (1988, p. 89) conclude that improvements in clinician
performance "were virtually always achieved through combinations of interventions rather than through isolated maneuvers."

For facilitators concerned with preventive care, the specific
combination of strategies varies from practice to practice. Administrative strategies are central to their role, but assisting practices
to implement patient-centered strategies (such as coaching patients to request indicated services and providing patient education literature) is also common. Professional education is more
often directed at nursing and other staff, but facilitators may also
provide physicians with educational resources and connect them
with experts in the field. An improved practice environment char-
acterized by a more active role for office staff and better office
organization may be more essential than increasing physician
knowledge, because physicians may already be well aware of the
desired guidelines.

Academic detailing is another strategy that combines interventions, usually professional education with administrative strategies such as feedback. Modeled on the approach of drug company representatives in which clinical experts work one-on-one with practicing physicians to influence prescribing patterns (Soumerai & Avorn, 1990), it appears to be efficacious in influencing physician prescribing practices (Soumerai & Avorn, 1987; Ray, Schaffner, & Federspiel, 1985). Its emphasis, however, differs from that of preventive care facilitators: It primarily addresses physician knowledge, rather than the practice environment. Its efficacy may rest on its ability to address all four stages of the application process described by Kaluzny et al. (1991) through limited contact with an expert. Recognition occurs prior to the detailing visit, because the community physician is already treating the condition. Identification that a specific systematic approach is necessary provides the main thrust of academic detailing visits. Reaching the Identification stage is aided by state-of-the-art knowledge and performance feedback delivered personally by an expert. The Implementation and Maintenance stages are reached after the detailing visit if the physician has been convinced that change is desirable and alters prescribing routines as a result. Such prescribing routines are followed internally by the physician and usually require no changes in the practice environment.

Most practice guidelines require changes that are more complex than just improving a prescribing pattern or increasing preventive services. In the middle of the spectrum of guideline dissemination approaches are those in which practice environment and physician knowledge must receive similar emphasis. For example, the insight that inflammation plays a central role in asthma lies at the foundation of current asthma guidelines (NHLBI, 1991) and distinguishes them from previous standards. Clinicians need to incorporate this new knowledge via professional education, but a second essential step is improving the practice environment so that office staff can support patients in self-management and physiologic monitoring as suggested in the guidelines. To our knowledge, this strategy to improve physician performance has not been tested in a randomized trial addressing a specific clinical condition.

Table 14.1 Alternative Dissemination Strategies to Promote Guideline Adoption by Practices at Various Stages of Readiness to Change

Readiness to Change Status	Minimal Strategy	Intensive Strategy
Recognition/Identification Stages	♦ Grand rounds ♦ Published guidelines	♦ Academic detailing ♦ Clinician workshop
Implementation/Maintenance Stages	♦ How-to manual ♦ Tool kit ♦ Periodic newsletters	♦ Facilitator ♦ Office staff workshop

Toward a Comprehensive Approach to Dissemination of Guidelines

Any practice guideline worth developing should have a formal dissemination plan attached. Table 14.1 describes minimal and intensive dissemination plans that apply to practices at various stages of readiness to change. Providing sufficient knowledge about the guideline will usually be a first step. Some physicians already recognize the importance of the clinical area and have identified the need for a more systematic approach, and their needs may be met by publication of the guidelines: If applying the guideline requires no support from the practice infrastructure, the physician may be able to make enduring changes him- or herself.

Practices that do not recognize the guideline service as part of their responsibility or that do not see the need for it may benefit from an academic detailing visit. For these, the need for further help with implementing a specific systematic approach will depend on its complexity and on the role of office staff.

If a change in the practice environment is required, external assistance may be needed along with attention to physician knowledge. This assistance could be provided by a facilitator, by training workshops for office staff, or perhaps by how-to manuals and kits that assist in modification of practice organization. Facilitators could be based in regional specialty societies, preventive advocacy groups, or academic medical centers as an adjunct to or substitute for some of their existing continuing medical education activities. A pilot test of one such program addressing cancer early detection is under way through the New Hampshire Division of the American Cancer Society.

The jump from newly published guidelines to physician performance often falls short. Dissemination plans and efforts deserve as much energy as the development of guidelines themselves. Attention to physicians' knowledge, their practice environments, and the readiness of practices to adopt guidelines may ease the jump from page to practice and perhaps even provide a bridge.

References

American Academy of Family Physicians Stop Smoking Program. (1987). *Patient stop smoking guide*. Kansas City, MO: American Academy of Family Physicians.

Berwick, D. M. (1989). Continuous improvement as an ideal in health care. *New England Journal of Medicine, 320*(1), 53-56.

Carney, P. A., Dietrich, A. J., Keller, A., Landgraf, J., & O'Connor, G. T. (1992). Tools, teamwork, and tenacity: An office system for cancer prevention. *Journal of Family Practice, 35*(4), 388-394.

Chomet, J., & Chomet, J. (1990). Cervical screening in general practice: A "new" scenario. *British Medical Journal, 300,* 1504-1506.

Cockburn, J., Ruth, D., Silagy, C., Dobbin, M., Reid, Y., Scollo, M., & Naccarella, L. (1992). Randomised trial of three approaches for marketing smoking cessation programmes to Australian general practitioners. *British Medical Journal, 304,* 691-604.

Coleman, J. S., Katz, E., & Menzel, H. (1966). *Medical innovation: A diffusion study*. Indianapolis, IN: Bobbs-Merrill.

Dietrich, A. J., O'Connor, G. T., Keller, A., Carney, P. A., Levy, D., & Whaley, F. S. (1992). Improving cancer early detection and prevention: A community practice randomized trial. *British Medical Journal, 304,* 687-691.

Eisenberg, J. M. (1986). Changing physicians' practice patterns. *Doctors' decisions and the cost of medical care* (pp 90-142). Ann Arbor, MI: Health Administration Press.

Ford, L. G., Hunter, C. P., Diehr, P., Frelick, R. W., & Yates, J. (1987). Effects of patient management guidelines on physician practice patterns: The community hospital oncology program experience. *Journal of Clinical Oncology, 5*(3), 504-511.

Fowler, G., Fullard, E., & Gray, M. (1992). Facilitating prevention in primary care [letter]. *British Medical Journal, 304,* 1177.

Fullard, E., Fowler, G., & Gray, M. (1984). Facilitating prevention in primary care. *British Medical Journal, 289,* 1585-1587.

Fullard, E., Fowler, G., & Gray, M. (1987). Promoting prevention in primary care: Controlled trial of low technology, low cost approach. *British Medical Journal, 204,* 1080-1082.

Gray, J. A. M., O'Dwyer, A., Fullard, E., & Fowler, G. (1987). Rent-an-Audit. *The Journal of the Royal College of General Practitioners, 37*, 177.

Greenfield, S., Kaplan, S. H., Ware, J. E., Martin, E., & Frank, H. (1988). Patient participation in medical care: Effects on blood sugar control, and quality of life in diabetes. *Journal of General Internal Medicine, 3*, 448-457.

Greer, A. L. (1988). The state of the art versus the state of the science. The diffusion of new medical technologies into practice. *International Journal of Technology Assessment in Health Care, 55*, 5-26.

Kaluzny, A. D., Harris, R. P., Strecher, V. J., Stearns, S., Qaqish, B., & Leininger, L. (1991). Prevention and early detection activities in primary care: New directions for implementation. *Cancer Detection and Prevention, 15*(6), 459-464.

Kottke, T. E., Solberg, L. I., Brekke, M. L., Conn, S. A., Maxwell, P., & Brekke, M. J. (1992). A controlled trial to integrate smoking cessation advice into primary care practice: Doctors helping smokers, round III. *Journal of Family Practice, 34*(6), 701-708.

Kritchevsky, S. B., Simmons, B. P. (1991). Continuous quality improvement. Concepts and applications for physician care. *Journal of the American Medical Association, 266*(13), 1817-1823.

Lomas, J., & Haynes, R. B. (1988). A taxonomy and critical review of tested strategies for the application of clinical practice recommendations: From "official" to "individual" clinical policy. In R. N. Battista & R. S. Lawrence (Eds.), Implementing preventive services. *American Journal of Preventive Medicine, 4*(4, Suppl.), 77-94.

Mant, D. (1992). Facilitating prevention in primary care. *British Medical Journal, 304*, 652-653.

McFadden, E. R., & Gilbert, I. A. (1992). Asthma. *New England Journal of Medicine, 327*(27) 1928-1937.

McPhee, S. J., Bird, J. A., Fordham, D., Rodnick, J. E., & Osborn, E. H. (1991). Promoting cancer prevention activities by primary care physicians: Results of a randomized controlled trial. *Journal of the American Medical Association, 266*(4), 538-544.

National Cancer Institute. (1987). *Working guidelines for early cancer detection: Rationale and supporting evidence to decrease mortality.* Bethesda, MD: National Institutes of Health.

National Cancer Institute Breast Cancer Screening Consortium. (1990). Screening mammography: A missed clinical opportunity? *Journal of the American Medical Association, 264*, 54-58.

National Heart, Lung, and Blood Institute. National Asthma Education Program Expert Panel Report. (1991). Guidelines for the diagnosis and management of asthma. *The Journal of Allergy and Clinical Immunology, 88*(3, Part 2), 425-534.

Pritchard, P., & Pritchard, J. (1992) *Developing teamwork in primary health care. A practical workbook.* Oxford: Oxford Medical Publications.

Ray, W. A., Schaffner, W., & Federspiel, C. F. (1985). Persistence of improvement in antibiotic prescribing in office practice. *Journal of the American Medical Association, 253*(12), 1774-1776.

Roberts, G. (Ed.). (1991). *Prevention in practice. A team approach.* Oxford: Radcliffe Medical Press.

Soumerai, S. B., & Avorn, J. (1987). Predictors of physician prescribing change in an educational experiment to improve medication use. *Medical Care, 25*(3), 210-221.

Soumerai, S. B., & Avorn, J. (1990). Principles of educational outreach ("academic detailing") to improve clinical decision making. *Journal of the American Medical Association, 263*(4), 540-556.

Tierney, W. M., Hui, S. L., & McDonald, C. J. (1986). Delayed feedback of physician performance versus immediate reminders to perform preventive care. Effects on physician compliance. *Medical Care, 25*(8), 659-666.

U.S. Department of Health and Human Services. (1992). *Prevention '91/'92: Federal programs and progress.* Washington, DC: Government Printing Office.

U.S. Preventive Services Task Force. (1989). *Guide to clinical preventive services.* Baltimore, MD: William & Wilkins.

15 Research Dissemination: The Practitioners' Perspective

MARILYN BOOKBINDER

Research dissemination is conceptualized as the initial step in a series of activities directed toward using research findings to answer a question in clinical practice. Changing the way practitioners practice, that is, policies and procedures, is an organizational process, which requires the commitment of both the practitioners delivering patient care and the administrators responsible for improving quality, cost-effective services. This chapter will focus on the practitioners' perspective, illustrating the conditions that hinder or facilitate their ability to implement research-based innovations. It describes three research utilization (RU) efforts, presenting examples of practitioners who sought to (a) solve a clinical problem, (b) promote prevention practices, and (c) improve hospital-wide quality of an important aspect of care.

Example 1:
Problem-Driven Research Utilization

In the two examples described here, nurses challenged traditional approaches to daily patient care. By questioning the basis for a procedure, they began the process of research utilization.

186

IV TUBING CHANGE

Hospital policy dictated changing IV tubing every 24 hours. Nurses on an active medical oncology unit questioned the basis for this practice, arguing that their immunocompromised patients were at increased risk for developing infections each time the tubing was changed. A telephone survey of other hospitals revealed a variation in practice from every 24 to every 72 hours and search of the literature showed that several studies (Band & Maki, 1979; Buxton et al., 1979; Gorbea, Snydman, Delaney, Stockman, & Martin, 1985; Josephson, Gombert, Sierra, Karanfil, & Tansino, 1985; Maki, Rhame, Mackel, & Bennett, 1976; U.S. Department of Health and Human Services, 1982) validated the safety of the less frequent changes. In fact, no differences were found in IV-associated bacteremias. On this unit no increased incidence in bacteremias was found after 6 months, and the policy was changed house-wide. This RU effort saved the institution more than $150,000 per year in IV tubing alone (Kenny, 1987).

FOLEY CATHETER CARE

Routine monitoring revealed nurses' low compliance with standard procedures for cleansing urinary catheters. Was this poor staff performance or simply another example of practitioners communicating to management that the standard procedure was no longer the "best"? Through the literature, nurses located six studies to confirm the research base that cleansing catheters with soap and water alone made no difference in the incidence of urinary tract infections (UTIs) than if they were washed with an antibacterial agent (Burke, Jacobson, Garibaldi, Conti, & Alling, 1983; Chawla, Clayton, & Stickler, 1988; Garibaldi, Burke, Butt, Miller, & Smith, 1980; Harvey, 1990; Kunin & Steele, 1985). These findings (Sauerland & Gaits, 1989) were presented to and approved by the hospital Quality Assurance (QA) and the Infectious Disease Departments, which continued to provide support by following the incidence of UTIs for the next 6 months on the two units proposing the practice change. With no documented differences on either unit, the new policy was implemented hospital-wide.

These examples serve to illustrate how research can be used to answer practice problems and provide the evidence needed to make a case for change. These RU efforts began during a time when the nursing shortage in the United States was at its peak and nurses were challenged to ration their time in the best way possible, so as to maintain the balance of providing quality, cost-effective patient care with limited resources. Nurses identified the areas where their efficiency could be improved. These were met with support by administration, who in turn identified an existing change process for the application of research findings, Quality Assessment. This mechanism paved the way for implementation of subsequent research-based practice changes (Bookbinder, 1992a, 1992b, 1993a, 1993b; Gaits et al., 1989).

Table 15.1 lists the parallel activities of the practitioner and administrator in the RU process. The importance of this complementary relationship in making organizational changes has been identified in four major projects in the field of nursing (Barnard, 1986; Funk, Tornquist, & Champagne, 1989; Horsley, Crane, & Bingle, 1978; Krueger, Nelson, & Wolanin, 1978). Implicit in the practitioner's role is the ability to act as the linkage agent, the person who connects research to users. Because the process is lengthy and complex, it requires practitioners to be educated in change theory and aspects of the research process (Goode & Bulechek, 1992). The role of the administrator is that of supplying support and assistance to linkage agents. Key to the process is the administrator's ability to identify mechanisms and persons to facilitate change efforts and place pressure on the organization's systems.

Example 2:
Prevention-Driven Research Utilization

This next example describes a study conducted by the author to investigate efforts of enterostomal therapy nurses (ETNs) to act as linkage agents in promoting the use of a skin risk assessment scale (SRAS) with known predictive value in identifying patients at risk for pressure sores (Bergstrom, Braden, Laguzza, & Holman, 1987;

Table 15.1 Practitioner and Administrator Roles in the Research
Utilization Process

Practitioner	Administrator
Clarify problem	Acknowledge relevance
Conduct literature review	Provide access to library
Obtain studies	Provide time
Critique studies	Provide education
Synthesize literature	Provide research expertise
Write proposal for change	Establish RU mechanism
Obtain approvals	Identify key opinion leaders
Implement innovation	Make project a priority
Evaluate change	Revise policy/procedure

Gosnell, 1973; Norton, McLaren, & Exton-Smith, 1962). Possible ETN linkage agents were surveyed, randomized, and stratified by 11 U.S. regions. An 88% response rate among hospital ETNs ($N = 263$) was achieved (Bookbinder, 1992a).

Two-thirds reported familiarity with the three research-based SRASs. Nearly half ($N = 113$) were using a nonresearch-based SRAS in their agency, with 48% using one of the three research-based scales. Only 9 nurses were using the SRAS exactly as developed by the authors: Most had made moderate to significant changes in the scale because they felt either a risk factor was missing or the scale did not "fit" their charting system. One third of hospitals were using an SRAS regularly, one third were trying to implement one, and the remainder had either reduced their efforts, discontinued them, or had never tried—reasons for this included a lack of administrative support for prevention practices and assistance in orchestrating the undertaking. Several administrators viewed the scales as overpredicting nursing care requirements and thus overspending.

Ease in using a scale and perceived benefits to patients ranked as the highest factors in facilitating the use of a prevention tool by nursing staff. Hindrances included nurses' lack of time and the perceived complexity of the scales available. Nearly 83% of ETNs not using a scale reported barriers to be overcome in their hospitals: structural or system changes, such as revising the patient record (33%); lack of support from middle management and administration (28%); and difficulty in selection of an SRAS (22%).

DISCUSSION

This study is consistent with the problem-driven examples described earlier and validates the need for administrative assistance in the RU process. It also suggests that training nurse specialists in the RU process may increase their ability to bring research into hospital practices, which can ultimately improve patient care.

Example 3:
Quality Improvement-Driven Research Utilization

The American Pain Society (APS) developed a set of standards entitled the Quality Assurance Standards for Acute Pain and Cancer Pain (Max et al., 1991). These standards were developed by experts in the field following a 2-year fact-finding period and were endorsed in the Agency for Health Care Policy and Research (AHCPR) guidelines for clinicians for acute pain management (Acute Pain Management Guideline Panel, 1992). In this third example, the first APS standard, "recognize and treat pain promptly," is examined using a continuous quality improvement (CQI) paradigm, to improve the quality of patient care in the area of pain management. Three principles of CQI guided the effort: redefining quality, designing data-based methods to constantly improve processes, and using statistical techniques.

The practitioners' first task was to define what quality means to the customer or recipient of the service or product. Although the ultimate customer is the patient, anyone involved in the process of delivering patient care can be a customer. Therefore departments and people can serve as providers/suppliers and customers in the same process (Miransky, 1993). For example, for a pharmacy to fill a prescription for pain medication, it must have a physician's order: when the pharmacy receives the order, it is the customer; when it fills the order, it is the supplier of the service to another customer—the nurse, who administers the dose. Problems in any part of the medication delivery process create a delay in patients receiving pain relief promptly.

Because customer needs are dynamic, practitioners need to assess customer satisfaction on a regular basis in order to assess the quality of services and ascertain whether improvement has occurred. In a pilot study to improve pain management practices, both nurses and patients on two study units were surveyed and independently chose "the time to administer medication" as the key quality process to examine.

The second principle is that, to achieve and maintain quality, processes must constantly be improved. In the paradigm of CQI, practitioners use scientific or data-based methods to study processes and measure improvement. Traditional problem-solving methods focus improvement efforts on extreme cases of a distribution, whereas CQI focuses on the most commonly occurring processes. The underlying assumption is that reducing variation in processes creates more control. As Deming (1986) notes: "A process that is in statistical control, stable, furnishes a rational basis for prediction for the results of tomorrow" (p. 350).

The third principle is the use of statistical techniques to study the processes for improvement. This study used a strategy called FOCUS-PDCA, an acronym meaning:

Find a process to improve,
Organize to improve the process,
Clarify current knowledge of the process,
Understand sources of process variation,
Select the process improvement.

Once a process improvement is selected,

Plan the improvement and continued data collection,
Do the improvement, data collection, and analysis,
Check and study the results,
Act to hold the gain and to improve the process.

The PDCA cycle for continuous improvement was first developed by Dr. Walter A. Shewhart and was popularized in Japan in the 1950s by Dr. W. Edwards Deming.

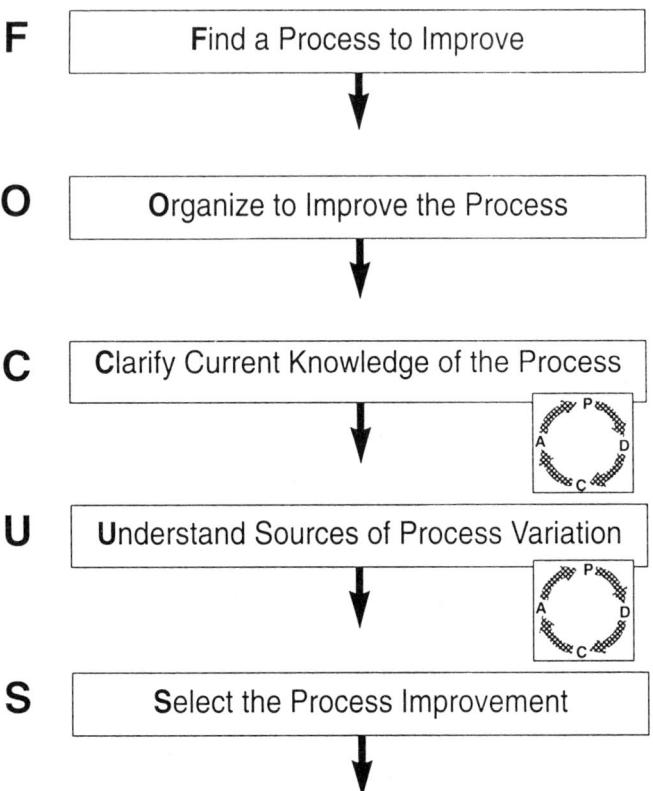

Figure 15.1. The FOCUS Strategy

SOURCE: FOCUS-PDCA is a registered trademark of Hospital Corporation of America. Used with permission.

Part of this section will walk through how the practitioners in our pain pilot example used the FOCUS strategy (see Figure 15.1) to examine a Key Quality Characteristic: Timeliness of Medication Delivery, that is, the time it takes from patient request for medication to administration of the dose by a nurse.

FOCUS—Practitioners first need to *find* a process to improve that is based on the needs of the customer and to identify both the boundaries of the process and the customers. The improvement of pain management was selected at our center for several reasons:

The organization's mission is to provide control of pain and suffering to cancer patients; two quality assurance studies had identified unrelieved pain as a priority concern for patients; and research-based guidelines and standards became available to assist clinicians in improving pain management practices in acute care settings.

FOCUS—Once boundaries were established, practitioners *organized* a team and planned the CQI effort. They needed to consider who had the process knowledge and who needed to be included on the team. Experts in pain management as well as all aspects of the medication delivery process and personnel with CQI expertise needed to be included: nurses, physicians, pharmacists, social workers, and a biostatistician.

FOCUS—Because no baseline data were available, practitioners needed to obtain information about the operation of the process. In this step, they *clarify* what is known about the process, both in-house and in the literature. It is here that research findings can be used to provide benchmarks or standards against which to compare results.

A flowchart mapping the entire medication delivery process was developed by team members to identify the correct process. This included prescribing, transcribing, prescription filling, and administering medication. The team then planned for data collection, first designing a tool that captured specific segments of the process: for example, the time to locate the patient's nurse and the nurse with narcotic keys, the time to prepare the medication, and delays in administering it once it was in hand. Using a systematic sampling technique, data collection took place over 2 days with the first 25 consecutive patients requesting pain medicine. Designated observers were assigned for the study period over the 48 hours to time the event. Because the purpose of this step was to provide baseline data, no improvements were implemented at this time.

Results from both patient surveys ($N = 364$) and nurses' time studies showed that the process was stable, with patients being medicated on average, less than 15 minutes. Improvement in the process requires further examination of the causes of variation.

FOCUS—The purpose of this next step is to gain an *understanding* of how the process varies over time and the causes of process variation. Practitioners judge whether the process is stable or whether it needs improvement. Is it meeting customer satisfaction and is there variation from special causes?

To help the staff examine the sources of variation, results were displayed by using Pareto charts, histograms, and control charts. Review of the data for the two units revealed that 30% of the variation on one unit was accounted for by delays in locating the narcotic keys, but this accounted for only 5% on the other unit. The time to locate the keys was significantly shorter on the unit where a "beeper" system was used in which the keys were attached to a beeper and the nurse needing them would page the number.

The goal here is to standardize the process as much as possible so that only one method is operating, thus reducing variation and increasing chances for more predictable outcomes.

Using the traditional approach, one would simply examine the cases where it took the longest time to get pain medication to the patient, then try to design strategies to encourage the people who are prescribing, filling the order, or administering medications to work more quickly. Although this approach may produce improvement for a few individuals, it does little to improve the daily process of medication delivery. Only one special case of a 45-minute delay was identified, where special filtered face masks required to enter the room of a patient on tuberculosis isolation precautions were out of stock.

FOCUS—*Select* the process improvement based on sources of variation in the process. This step focuses on answering the question, "What changes can be made to improve the process?"

Because the largest variation on one unit occurred in locating the narcotic keys, discussion centered around adopting the beeper system used so successfully on the other unit. Other causes of delay and possible solutions were also discussed: needing to call the physician to renew or change medication orders and being called to tend another patient at the time of the request.

PDCA—*Plan* the improvement. Changes being made to the process are carefully planned by the team before they are introduced. Getting approvals, communicating with key people, and planning education and data collection procedures are addressed in this phase. In the example described here, an improvement effort is being planned for the pilot units that will involve an innovative computerized system for storing, retrieving, and re-

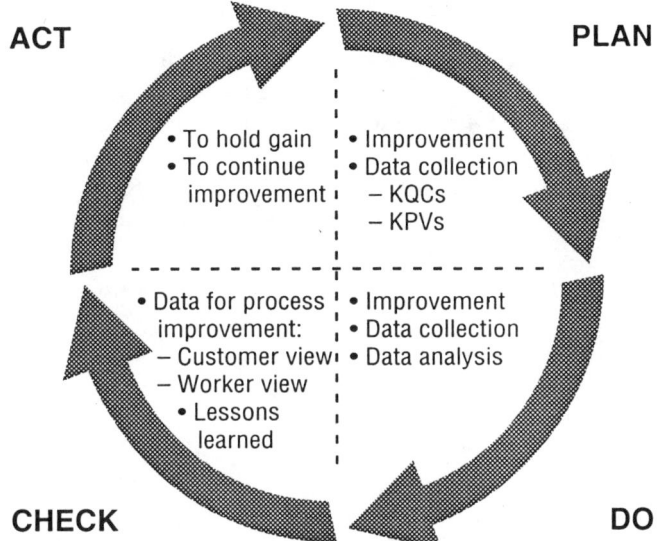

Figure 15.2. The PCDA Strategy

SOURCE: FOCUS-PDCA is a registered trademark of Hospital Corporation of America. Used with permission.

cording narcotics. This system eliminates the need for narcotic keys and reduces the time spent on documentation by nurses, as well as other administrative and patient features.

PDCA—*Do* the improvement process. The plan is carried out, preferably small, noting any changes that occur during implementation. In this example, the new system will be tested on the two pilot units, and data collection will be repeated using the same tool as before the implementation of the computerized system.

PDCA—*Check* and examine results. This step examines what was learned and seeks to understand any unexpected results. Our new data will be compared against previous results. (Of course, different types of delays may occur with the new system and will need to be examined.)

PDCA—*Act* to hold the gain and continue to improve the process. If our results show improvement, then computerization will be implemented on these units and considered house-wide. If unsuccessful, reexamination of the improvement process is needed (see Figure 15.2).

The team returns to the F (FOCUS) step to discuss boundaries for the next improvement process. Members may agree to study another segment of the same process (timeliness of medication administration) or redirect their attention to a different one. Besides serving to focus the team, the FOCUS-PDCA framework keeps members from feeling overwhelmed and keeps their improvement efforts manageable.

Summary

The first set of examples illustrates how a traditional hospital mechanism, quality assurance, facilitated practitioners' use of research findings to answer practice problems. Nurses' mastery in formulating a research base along with assistance from administration to lift organizational barriers, were keys to successful policy changes.

The second example, prevention-driven RU, describes some of the practical problems faced by one group of specialty nurses when using an assessment scale with known predictability. Although half of the total sample reported using such a scale, nearly half changed the original tool or created their own. Only four reported evaluation efforts, and none reported a continuing feedback mechanism where improvement could be measured.

In the third example, health professionals used a continuous quality improvement paradigm to bring research into their daily practice. Because those affected by the change must be part of it, perspectives from all customers (practitioners and patients) are considered. Administrative support is integral to examining the processes of delivering patient care and using results to improve outcomes. Organizations that place value on continuous improvement methods and view the application of knowledge as a means to achieve quality can facilitate the dissemination of research into practice more effectively than those who do not. Within this paradigm, teams representing various disciplines have the opportunity to pool their knowledge and expertise to produce a more comprehensive research base upon which to make practice decisions.

References

Acute Pain Management Guideline Panel. (1992). *Acute pain management: Operative medical procedures and trauma. Clinical practice guidelines* (AHCPR Pub. No. 920032). Rockville, MD: U.S. Department of Health and Human Services, Public Health Service, Agency for Health Care Policy and Research.

Band, J. D., & Maki, D. G. (1979). Safety of changing intravenous delivery systems of longer than 24 hour intervals. *Annals of Internal Medicine, 90,* 173-178.

Barnard, K. E. (1986, May-June). Research utilization: The clinician's role. *American Journal of Maternal and Child Nursing, 11,* 224.

Bergstrom, N., Braden, B., Laguzza, A., & Holman, V. (1987). The Braden scale for predicting pressure sore risk. *Nursing Research, 36*(4), 205-210.

Bookbinder, M. (1992a). Nurse linkage agents' efforts to facilitate the use of a research-based innovation. *Dissertation Abstracts International.* (University Microfilms No. 92-37, 737)

Bookbinder, M. (1992b). Research: What's in it for you? *Nursing Spectrum, 4*(2), 8.

Bookbinder, M. (1992c). Searching for solutions. *Nursing Spectrum, 4*(13), 10.

Bookbinder, M. (1993a). Making research work for you. *Nursing Spectrum, 5*(2), 8.

Bookbinder, M. (1993b). Research, practice, quality care. *Nursing Spectrum, 5*(21), 7-16.

Burke, J., Jacobson, R., Garibaldi, M., Conti, M., & Alling, D. (1983). Evaluation of daily meatal care with poly-antibiotic ointment in prevention of urinary catheter-associated bacteriuria. *Journal of Urology, 129,* 331-334.

Buxton, A. E., Highsmith, A. K., Garner, J. S., West, M., Stamm, W. E., Dixon, R. E., & McGowan, J. E. (1979). Contamination of intravenous infusion fluid: Effects of changing administration sets. *Annals of Internal Medicine, 90,* 764-768.

Chawla, J. C., Clayton, C. L., & Stickler, D. J. (1988). Antiseptics in the long-term urological management of patients by intermittent catheterization. *British Journal of Urology, 62,* 289-294.

Deming, W. E. (1986). *Out of the crisis.* Cambridge: MIT Center For Advanced Engineering Study.

Funk, S. G., Tornquist, E. M., & Champagne, M. T. (1989). A model for improving the dissemination of research. *Western Journal of Nursing Research, 11*(3), 361-367.

Gaits, V., Nuscher, R., Kaplow, R., Bru, G., Belcher, A., Brown, M. H., & Bookbinder, M. (1989). Unit-based research forums: A model for the clinical nurse specialist to promote research. *Clinical Nurse Specialist, 3*(2), 60-65.

Garibaldi, R., Burke, J., Butt, M., Miller, W., & Smith, C. (1980). Meatal colonization and catheter-associated bacteriuria. *The New England Journal of Medicine, 303,* 316-318.

Gorbea, H. F., Snydman, D. R., Delaney, A., Stockman, J., & Martin, W. J. (1985). Intravenous tubing with burettes can be safely changed at 48-hour intervals. *Journal of the American Medical Association, 251,* 2112-2115.

Goode, C., & Bulechek, G. M. (1992). Research utilization in a practice setting. *Journal of Nursing Quality Care* (A special report), 27-35.

Gosnell, D. J. (1973). An assessment to identify pressure sores. *Nursing Research, 22,* 55-59.

Harvey, S. (1980). Antiseptics and disinfectants, fungicides, ectoparasiticides. In L. S. Goodman & A. Gilman (Eds.), *The pharmacological basis of therapeutics* (8th ed.), (pp. 964-987). New York: Macmillan.

Horsley, J. A., Crane, J., & Bingle, J. D. (1978). Research utilization as an organizational process. *The Journal of Nursing Administration, 8,* 4-6.

Josephson, A., Gombert, M. E., Sierra, M. F., Karanfil, L. V., & Tansino, G. F. (1985). The relationship between intravenous fluid contamination and the frequency of tubing replacement. *Infection Control, 6,* 267-370.

Kenny, S. (1987, January). *Frequency of changing IV tubing.* Paper presented at Hospital Quality Assurance meeting, Memorial Sloan-Kettering Cancer Center, NY.

Krueger, J., Nelson, A. H., & Wolanin, M. O. (1978). *Nursing research: Development, collaboration and utilization.* Germantown, MD: Aspen Systems.

Kunin, C., & Steele, C. (1985). Culture of the surfaces of urinary catheters to sample urethral flora and study the effect of antimicrobial therapy. *Journal of Clinical Microbiology, 21,* 902-908.

Maki, D. G., Rhame, F. S., Mackel, D. C., & Bennett, J. V. (1976). Nationwide epidemic of septicemia caused by contaminated intravenous products. *American Journal of Medicine, 60,* 471-485.

Max, M. B., Donovan, M., Portenoy, R. K., Cleeland, C. S., Ready, L. B., Carr, D. B., Edwards, W. T., Simmonds, M. A., & Evans, W. O. (1991). American Pain Society quality assurance standards for relief of acute pain and cancer pain. In M. Bond, J. E. Charlton, & C. J. Woolf (Eds.), *Proceedings of the VIth World Congress on Pain* (pp. 185-190). Amsterdam: Elsevier.

Miransky, J. (1993, January). *Principles of quality improvement.* Paper presented at Hospital Quality Assurance meeting, Memorial Sloan-Kettering Cancer Center, NY.

Norton, D., McLaren, R., & Exton-Smith, A. B. (1962). *An investigation of geriatric nursing problems in hospitals.* London: Churchill Livingstone.

Sauerland, C., & Gaits, V. (1987, April). *Noneffectiveness of daily mental care: A review of the literature.* Paper presented at Hospital Quality Assurance meeting, Memorial Sloan-Kettering Cancer Center, NY.

U. S. Department of Health and Human Services (PHS). (1982). *Guidelines for prevention of intravenous therapy-related infections.* Atlanta, GA: Centers for Disease Control.

16 Using Research and Evaluation Results in Health Services Policy Making

VIVEK GOEL
C. DAVID NAYLOR

Despite the enormous increase over the past two decades in research activities devoted to evaluating health care, there has been inconsistent success in translation of research results into health care practice and policy. The issues of implementing research findings in clinical practice have been reviewed in earlier chapters, and elsewhere by Lomas and colleagues (Grilli & Lomas, 1994; Lomas, 1991; Lomas & Haynes, 1988). This chapter focuses instead on the interface between research and health policy development. We explore barriers to implementation, and potential solutions that will help policy makers and researchers interact more effectively.

Types of Studies and Results

Two phases of health care research are commonly described: *efficacy*—whether an intervention works in ideal circumstances, and *effectiveness*—whether it works in usual practice (Tugwell, Bennett, Sackett, & Haynes, 1985). Researchers are also concerned with *efficiency*—the relative value of the intervention, usually tallied as some ratio of inputs and outputs or efforts and yields (Tugwell et al., 1985).

These types of evaluations are applicable to the entire gamut of health care interventions. This includes not only treatments of patients with disease, but also public health interventions (e.g., health promotion strategies), organizational interventions (e.g., changes in structures or reimbursement of health care providers), and interventions to change how treatments are used (e.g., dissemination of treatment guidelines or education programs for health care providers).

Methodological research explores the ways that evaluations can best be carried out. Thus, an epistemological distinction can be made between health care evaluation—the application of evaluation methods to health care—and methodological research concerned with evaluative techniques. No sharply drawn border separates these two areas of activity. Moreover, a phase of research may be needed in the first instance to lay the methodological groundwork that allows more practical or policy-oriented investigation and analysis to be undertaken.

End Users of Research Results

An idealized view of clinical research assumes that results from studies are taken up by practitioners and incorporated routinely into the care of patients. A key lesson of health services research has been the extent to which practice patterns in all areas of medicine depart from this idealized view. By the same token, one cannot assume that policy makers and opinion leaders will absorb and implement the results of evaluative research. Simply contemplating the range of potential end users highlights the magnitude of the "research transfer" problem. Potential end users include professionals in clinical leadership positions (e.g., chiefs of staff, medical directors, heads of specialty societies, etc.); hospital administrators; policy makers in public agencies, such as bureaucrats and politicians; policy makers in so-called private governments, such as licensing and regulatory bodies for health professionals; and consumers of health care, either individually or organized into advocacy groups. Research results of all types are also used by information providers such as the news media.

Policy Development Cycle

Many authors have described the process of policy development (e.g., see Crichton, 1981, pp. 318-320; Pal, 1987). The first step is issue identification. Issues may be brought to attention by patients, providers, advocacy and interest groups, and politicians or bureaucrats. Health care issues are also sometimes raised by researchers or evaluators. A recurrent problem in any publicly funded health care system is the process whereby issues are identified as worthy of attention. Items that are newsworthy usually galvanize political attention. Thus an agenda of longer term initiatives may be derailed by political pressures and interest group lobbying. Evaluation and research can be useful at the issue identification stage in obtaining information on the impact of the issue, a process often referred to as needs assessment.

Once an issue is selected, the next two steps involve identifying programs or interventions to deal with that issue, and selecting a course of action. The more political the decision-making process, the greater the number of potential players there will be. Health care research can again make key contributions at this stage by offering data on the efficacy, effectiveness, and efficiency of the proposed responses to the issue of concern.

Finally, once a program or intervention is implemented, evaluation can play a role in ensuring that the program is set in motion as proposed and in monitoring it to ensure that it operates effectively and efficiently. This process can also be used to ensure that the program is responsive to a changing environment in ways that optimize ongoing effectiveness and efficiency.

Because ministries of health are themselves perceived to be stakeholders with positions to defend, information provided by governments is sometimes challenged by the media and interest groups. Even evaluation consultants hired by governments may be viewed skeptically. Analyses and evaluations that provide political insulation against incendiary issues are perhaps best performed by those who, traditionally, have been least likely to do so in a timely fashion—academic health care researchers.

Although evaluation and research have a role to play in each of the steps described above, policies are developed with an eye to many inputs other than evidence per se. For example, senior policy makers will be influenced by interest group pressures, lobbyists, royal commissions and other official reports (which may or may not hew to evidence), unofficial or anecdotal research, public opinion polls, and advice from the bureaucracy. This mixture of inputs is then blended with caucus politics, personalities and ideologies, congressional or parliamentary exchanges, committee dynamics, and media coverage. The power of research and evaluation to drive such a political process is obviously limited. These and other barriers to evidence-based policy making are reviewed below.

Barriers to Using the Results of Research and Evaluation

Barriers that attenuate the influence of research and evaluation in health services policy making can be grouped in three categories: those arising with the research and evaluation process, those arising in the health care system itself, and those arising because of the characteristics of policy makers and the pressures to which they are subject.

PROBLEMS WITH RESEARCH/EVALUATION

Timeliness of research and evaluation is a fundamental problem in its applicability. Most research takes a long time to complete, and research results are often not available until after a policy decision has already had to be made. This is particularly germane in the area of new technology. By the time researchers complete the assessment of a new technology in a form that can be used by policy makers, a whole new generation of technologies may exist to replace the one that has been assessed. Rather than wait for primary data collection to provide the needed information, evaluators and researchers can draw on existing data, such as hospital discharge abstracts or claims databases. These administrative data, however, are often in a form that cannot be readily used by researchers (e.g., critical variables are missing, or there are restrictions on access to certain fields of data for confidentiality reasons). These data are also observational and do not offer the definitive evidence about efficacy that arises from randomized controlled trials.

Policy makers, as well as the researchers or evaluators providing advice to them, must also deal with major gaps in the health care knowledge base. Health care providers must often make decisions of a probabilistic nature when diagnosing disease and choosing treatments. This lack of certainty at the clinical level is reflected in the incomplete knowledge base that is used to formulate clinically relevant policies. Because inferences must be made on the basis of incomplete evidence, interpretive conflict among researchers is not uncommon.

The technical nature of research results itself poses an inherent barrier to comprehension by policy makers, and academically rebarbative styles add to the confusion. As quantitative methods and models become more commonplace, the translation problems are compounded.

Conflicting results that arise in health care research are a further source of frustration to decision makers. In many instances, however, this is due to legitimate reasons related to subtle differences in the populations studied, interventions, outcome measures, and analytical techniques. Differences also occur by chance alone, because studies rely on probabilistic inference. Partly in response to the random variations in results of otherwise similar studies, meta-analysis has become popular in the health care field (Sacks, Berrier, Reitman, Ancona-Berk, & Chalmers, 1987). Meta-analyses aggregate the results of multiple studies and are particularly valuable adjuncts for policy making. The research literature amply documents the potential pitfalls in meta-analysis, however. Results from meta-analyses can also be confusing for the reader who lacks methodological training.

Even when evidence from a number of well-conducted studies is more or less consistent, interpretive disagreements among researchers can arise. This is sometimes attributable to different disciplinary backgrounds or to ideological differences. Indeed, much of health care research is value-laden. Selection of research questions, study subjects, implementation of interventions, control variables, and methods of analysis are all steps at which values can shape the scientific enterprise.

Tensions also arise between the persons implementing and running programs, and evaluators or researchers. Program personnel have a responsibility to ensure that the program runs smoothly and delivers the services that it should and will tend to be intellectually and emotionally committed to the program. The evaluators who wish to collect data and observe the program may not only temporarily interfere with its smooth operation, but, more fundamentally, pose an implicit threat to all those associated with it.

Last but by no means least, some research findings may simply be uninteresting for policy makers. Much of the clinical research enterprise in industrialized nations addresses questions that appear at first glance to be almost willfully irrelevant. Academic researchers, in particular, cherish their independence to do curiosity-oriented work. Their approach in general is top-down: Researchers generate ideas and innovations, and expect that the fruits of their labors will diffuse through the system. In the absence of a more needs-oriented approach to generating questions for evaluative and methodological research, some of the output of the academic research establishment ends up appearing as a set of solutions in search of a problem.

PROBLEMS WITH THE HEALTH SERVICES SYSTEM

The health services system itself throws up several barriers to the ready application of research results in health policy development. Reimbursement systems for health care providers in most industrialized nations do not offer specific incentives for them to participate in—or lead—evaluation activities. Training of providers in evaluative methods is limited and may actually be counterproductive. In particular, the concept of teaching "critical appraisal" of the clinical research literature is now internationally popular in undergraduate and/or postgraduate programs for clinicians. This threatens to become a new variant on yesteryear's theme of the omniscient clinician and cannot be construed as a substitute for policies and systems to promote evidence-based and efficient practice patterns.

In institutional settings, such as hospitals and large clinics, constrained budgets and the need for patient throughput generate incentives to ensure efficient operations. Thus the importance of evaluation is enhanced. In Canadian hospitals, however, resources for this type of activity are not built into base budgets, and hospitals developing evaluation units must either raise funds through other sources, or commit internal resources that might otherwise go to patient care and related activities. District health councils have limited financial resources to undertake major evaluative activities and little authority to translate research findings into policy making at the district or regional level.

More generally, the structure of the Canadian health care system is not optimal for evidence-based policy implementation. Physicians and hospitals operate as state-dependent contractors—the former as private fee-for-service practitioners in a public insurance system; the latter as private nonprofit corporations funded largely by annual allocations from provincial health ministries (Naylor, 1992b). Health ministries have therefore tended to function as insurers for physician services and funders for general hospital care, without assuming a strong management role. Indeed, control of the delivery system itself is highly decentralized, with ongoing inadequacies in the regionalization or rationalization of services (Ugnat & Naylor, 1993). As ministries move to manage the system in a more active fashion, they repeatedly bump up against the difficulties of setting policies on a centralized basis for a decentralized system with moderate to marked regional variations in practice patterns. Providers and patients may lobby to bring services to a higher common denominator, rather than weigh the trade-offs necessary in a sector with limited resources.

Devolution of pooled hospital funds and even physician billing budgets to regional health authorities is being touted as a vehicle to promote more explicit policy and program trade-offs. With enhanced local accountability for "service purchasing" decisions comes a greater potential for evidence-based debate about funding priorities. Although some Canadian provinces are now moving to regionalized budgetary envelopes, the evaluative infrastructures to support regionalization are underdeveloped. Regional health authorities in the National Health Service of the United Kingdom, by way of contrast, have entered into a variety of arrangements to obtain evaluative services that will guide policy making and spending decisions.

PROBLEMS WITH THE POLICY PROCESS

Behind the issue of how research evidence is used in policy making is the basic issue of how policy is made. As described above, policy development is a complex and quasirational process. We discuss here a few of its aspects that are related to the use of research results.

The role of lobbies and interest groups has been well documented in health policy development (Taylor, 1978). Health care providers form especially strong lobby groups. This group includes not only health professionals, but also hospitals and other institutions, as well as manufacturers of drugs and medical equipment. Many of these groups are the source of research that has an impact on policy decisions. Important influence is also exerted by advocacy groups concerned with specific conditions such as cancer or cardiovascular disease. These disease-advocacy groups take an active role in fund-raising and may support research, public education, and specialized patient services. Disease-based interest groups are also called upon to summarize and present results of research to policy makers.

Providers and advocacy groups often market their viewpoints to the general public rather than to policy makers, on the reasonable assumption that elected politicians are susceptible to public pressure. Public perception, in turn, is molded in large part by the news media. The challenges of communicating research results, some of which are described in other chapters, are further complicated when dealing with the media and with the biases that interest groups bring to the interpretation of research for public consumption.

Even where the requisite research findings are synthesized and translated into useable concepts, bureaucratic obstacles arise to their utilization within many public service organizations. Civil servants are buffeted by the backlash from interest groups with each policy change or innovation. This phenomenon is especially intense in unitary public health systems such as exist in most industrialized countries. In an internationally generalizable description, Evans et al. (1989) pointed out that public payment sets government up as the target for all stakeholders, allowing "orchestrated outrage" rather than the "diffuse distress" that characterizes American providers facing challenges from a multiplicity of private and public payers. In a public system, research can be regarded as a catalyst for unwelcome change, including increased demand for service delivery and payment at a time when dollars are scarce.

Given the many other factors inherent in policy making, expert advisors may tend to pick and choose among studies or subanalyses within studies for data that support a politically expedient viewpoint or goal. These selection biases are not necessarily the result of premeditation: Bureaucrats may only become aware of, or be in contact with, evaluators and researchers sympathetic to their own interests.

Ultimately responsibility for health policy decisions in Western democratic societies rests with elected officials. These officials usually do not have a background in health services research and tend to rely on bureaucrats and other professional advisors to distill and interpret evidence. Both elected officials and advisers are also constrained by time pressures and may not have the luxury to seek and act upon all relevant data. Decisions and policies may therefore appear illogical to those outside the system, but such criticism ignores the manner in which decisions must be made, including the complex blend of political and evidentiary inputs that lead to a final policy.

All things considered, it is not surprising that public commissions and task forces have been a common recourse in every country for health policy makers faced with difficult decisions. The commission or task force can operate outside the hurly-burly of the political arena. It can hear out the interested parties, distill stakeholder opinions, build up a profile and relationship with the media, contract with experts to undertake primary research or to synthesize extant research findings, and ultimately provide policy advice of a high quality. Few commissions or task forces, however, make their cases with such force or moral authority that decision makers are bound to implement their recommendations. The recommendations themselves become another input to the policy-making process, and the complex cycle continues.

Possible Solutions

How can evaluation researchers and research results contribute more to policy making?

First and foremost, the research agenda must be made more relevant to stakeholder needs and policy makers' priorities. In Canada this concern has led to the creation of mission-oriented health service research groups tied variously to government alone or to government and various providers or stakeholders. In addition, individual agencies, such as major hospitals, are also moving to create evaluation units concerned with the appropriateness and efficiency of services provided internally. This gives the policy makers in the hospital—the senior management and clinical leaders—immediate access to evidence about practice patterns. Eventually, it will be important for all health science centers and university-based evaluation groups to develop a more needs-oriented approach to research, while sustaining the traditional curiosity-driven research carried out by academic investigators. We emphasize the need for balance; top-flight academic researchers will never be drawn to an agency where their investigative energies are entirely at the beck and call of stakeholders and governments.

The relevance of peer-reviewed research must also be addressed. For example, Canadian agencies expend much more effort in ensuring the methodological standards of grant submissions than in assessing their relevance and service delivery implications. Again, we acknowledge the need to sustain curiosity-driven academic research. In a time of constrained resources, however, managers of peer-reviewed grant review processes must ensure that relevant research is conducted. In the United States these concerns have led to the creation of the Agency for Health Care Policy and Research, dedicated specifically to the pursuit of relevant topics in health services research.

Second, researchers and policy makers must speak a common language. Researchers in practice and in training must be made aware of how research results are applied and used (or not used). Researchers are not adept at putting findings forward in plain terms, and some academics appear to seek shelter behind jargon and careful qualifiers in an attempt to evade responsibility for actions that might flow from their findings! For their part, bureaucracies must develop the in-house "translation" capacity so that policy decisions can be made with due attention to evidence. Users of research results need basic education on the pitfalls in research and some training in how to interpret results (Chambers, Stoddart, & Sullivan, 1983). Political realities mean that quasirational inputs must always play a role in policy making. Understanding of evaluation methods on the part of key bureaucrats is, however, a potential safeguard that will promote a more evidence-based approach to decision making.

In both respects we note a serious training deficiency. Traditionally Canada has produced health administration specialists with a managerial orientation, and epidemiologists with a clinical or population focus. There is no training program oriented to preparing health service researchers who can pinpoint the gaps between research evidence and practice patterns, or to preparing research-oriented managers who will be adept at translating research results for policy makers or at formulating draft policies for elected officials.

Third, there needs to be a general acceptance by health care providers and other interest groups that the totality of research evidence can and should be used to guide policy making wherever possible. Stakeholders are accustomed to using evidence selectively to legitimize group ends, thereby casting policy makers in the role of a jury weighing competing arguments. Researchers contribute to the polarization by talking to each other, rather than to the wider circle of persons who might leaven their academic preoccupations with common sense and practical insights. Seminars and workshops that bring together researchers, stakeholders, and policy makers could play a part in creating the necessary evidence-based dialogue about how and where the health-care system should evolve.

Fourth, a close look at current reimbursement mechanisms for health care professionals and institutions is required to generate incentives for the adoption of the relevant results of research. Beyond the concept of reimbursement per se, it may be appropriate to experiment with alternative funding systems that place providers for a region under a budgetary umbrella, with free flow of information about practice patterns and outcomes to help drive more rational resource allocation.

Fifth and finally, an inventory of relevant research activities and expertise must be maintained, with some form of clearinghouse function to ensure that policy makers know who the experts are and what relevant research is being performed or could be performed in short order to meet decisional needs. Encouragingly, in Canada such an initiative is now on the agenda of an Advisory Committee to the Conference of Deputy Ministers of Health.

Afterthought

The history of Canadian health care teaches us that "social change is inevitable and institutional progress possible, but human nature is wonderfully intransigent" (Naylor, 1992a, p. 12). We remain profoundly cognizant of the fact that policy making, like politics, is in some measure the art of managing intransigence. The role of research and researchers is to leaven policy making with evaluation evidence so that the possibilities for change will be better understood and the potential for progress more readily achieved.

References

Chambers, L. W., Stoddart, G. L., & Sullivan, B. (1983). Continuing education for health professionals and administrators: Workshops on becoming a critical user of health care research. *Canadian Journal of Public Health, 74*, 29-34.

Crichton, A. (1981). *Health policy making*. Ann Arbor, MI: Health Administration Press.

Evans, R. G., Lomas, J., Barer, M. L., Labelle, R. J., Fooks, C., Stoddart, G. L., Anderson, G. M., Seeny, D., Gafni, A., Torrence, G. W., & Tholl, W. G. (1989). Controlling health expenditures: The Canadian reality. *New England Journal of Medicine, 320*(9), 571-577.

Grilli, R., & Lomas, J. (1994). Evaluating the message: The relationship between compliance rate and the subject of a practice guideline, *Medical Care, 32*(3), 202-213.

Lomas, J. (1991). Words without actions? The production, dissemination and impact of consensus recommendations. *Annual Reviews of Public Health, 12*, 41-65.

Lomas, J., & Haynes, R. B. (1988). A taxonomy and critical review of tested strategies for the application of clinical practice recommendations: From "official" to "individual" clinical policy. In R. N. Battista & R. S. Lawrence

(Eds.), Implementing preventive services. *American Journal of Preventive Medicine, 4*(4, Suppl.), 77-94.

Naylor, C. D. (Ed.). (1992a). *Canadian health care and the state: A century of evolution.* Montreal: McGill-Queen's University Press.

Naylor, C. D. (1992b). The Canadian health care system: A model for America to emulate? *Health Economics, 1,* 19-37.

Pal, L. A. (1987). *Public policy analysis: An introduction.* Toronto: Methuen.

Sacks, H. S., Berrier, J., Reitman, D., Ancona-Berk, V. A., & Chalmers, T. C. (1987). Meta-analyses of randomized controlled trials. *New England Journal of Medicine, 316,* 450-455.

Taylor, M. G. (1978). *Health insurance and Canadian public policy: The seven decisions that created the Canadian health insurance system.* Montreal: McGill-Queen's University Press.

Tugwell, P., Bennett, K. J., Sackett, D. L., & Haynes, R. B. (1985). The measurement iterative loop. *Journal of Chronic Diseases, 38,* 339-351.

Ugnat, A. M., & Naylor, C. D. (1993). *Small area variations in the use of coronary surgery in Ontario, 1981-1989* (Working Paper Series No. 002). North York: Institute for Clinical Evaluative Sciences in Ontario.

Appendix:
Tips on Dealing With the Media

SHARON LINDENBURGER

As Peter Desbarats observes in Chapter 6 of this volume, "The Media and the Dissemination of Research," medicine and journalism are "two solitudes," each with different agendas and priorities concerning how information is conveyed to the public. Many journalists, even those covering medical issues, do not have a scientific background, and most scientists are not taught strategies to help them communicate the important aspects of their discipline to nonscientists.

Yet, as Desbarats points out, the public relies heavily on the media for the latest information on medicine and health care. He aptly arrives at the conclusion that "the failure of media to adequately cover science, medicine, and health issues directly affects the ability of individuals to protect themselves from disease and to support institutional changes that would enable society to improve the systems that promote and protect our well-being."

Because the media by and large are always after "a good story" and most reporters really do want to get things right, an important part of the bridge-building needed to connect these two solitudes must come from scientists gaining a greater comfort level and confidence in dealing with the media. If, as Desbarats says, the

213

media need to do a better job of covering health issues, then medical professionals who have health care findings of interest also need to do a better job of communicating to the public through the media.

When disseminating information aimed at the general public, the scientist should set aside his or her "scientific mind-set" and think like a lay person. One strategy I have used in working with medical scientists involved in leading-edge biomedical research is to ask them to imagine they are talking to a Grade 11 science class about their research and its potential significance for health care. That is, how would you describe to 16-year-old adolescents what you do and why you do it? How would you hold their attention? What happens is interesting—verbs become more active, the sentences shorter, colorful anecdotes emerge, the conversational style relaxes. And the result is a reader-friendly article or interview that does convey the essence of the scientist's research or point of view in terms the public will understand and enjoy hearing about.

This appendix discusses some strategies for approaching or responding to the news media. The areas considered include how to issue press releases, dealing with on-air or press interviews, and responding to patients who are influenced by what they read or hear in the news.

Contacting the Media

The most common methods chosen by medical scientists who want to make the results of their research known in the public arena are to contact newspapers or television stations by telephone, or to issue a news release. I strongly recommend the latter. When you convey news by telephone, you are handing over a snippet of your story for further fleshing out by the publication or network staff (if they are interested), and leaving it totally up to the reporter to come up with the relevant questions. But with a news release, you have the advantage of supplying something concrete in writing; of ensuring ahead of time that the information you are providing is accurate; and of identifying its source. Reporters and editors appreciate a well-written, interesting news release because it gives them a solid basis to begin constructing a newsworthy story.

Of course, a rambling news release that lacks focus will probably result in the story being consigned to the garbage. A clear, concise one is no guarantee the story will end up being covered (no matter how interesting researchers think their subjects are, editors do not always agree), but it will greatly increase your odds—not only of being covered but of being covered accurately. Following are some suggestions of how to achieve this.

THE CHARACTERISTICS OF A GOOD NEWS RELEASE

1. Put yourself in the position of the average reader or TV viewer, and ask yourself from that perspective: What is the most interesting or important aspect of this story? Include this in the "lead"—your first paragraph. Another strategy for arriving at a good lead is to imagine discussing your topic at a social gathering. What part of it would arouse the most interest or discussion? What would get people talking?

2. Follow journalism's classic "five w's"—who, what, where, when, and why—and don't forget "how." Only the most vital of these should be part of your lead; the others can be touched on further down.

3. Use the active voice, not the passive. Wherever possible, use the present tense instead of the past.

4. Avoid using the jargon of your discipline: Translate clinical terms to words or phrases familiar to the layperson. For example, do not say "cholecystectomy": say "gall bladder surgery."

5. Do not load a news release with a large number of statistics. Quote only the most important ones—for example, "Stress is a significant concern in 60%-70% of patients' visits to family physicians."

6. Include good conversational quotes. If you are the spokesperson for the research project, make up a direct quote for yourself. Write it as dialogue, as if you were actually speaking to someone. If you are quoting someone else, do it in the same way. (Example: "The results of this study will have enormous implications for how family doctors practice across Canada," says Dr. I. Care of the University of Ontario.) The sense of someone talking contributes to the human quality of the release and moves the story forward.

7. Keep both paragraphs and sentences relatively short. The news release should fit onto one page. Think in terms of seven or eight short paragraphs, maximum.

8. At the end, write something like "For more information on _____ contact Dr. I. Care at _____." Sometimes you can name more than one contact, but do not name more than three.

THE FORMAT OF A NEWS RELEASE

Your news release should be:

1. Neatly typed or printed on 8½" x 11" paper.
2. Free of typos or grammatical errors.
3. Datelined with the name of the city and the date the news is released. Place the words "FOR IMMEDIATE RELEASE" at the top, above the headline.
4. Readily identifiable—use letterhead paper that identifies your office or institution, and ideally includes a printed headline such as "Newslink" or "Medialink."
5. Headlined in uppercase letters. Create a short title or headline that will immediately tell editors what the release is about—for example, MORE FAMILY DOCTORS ARE MAKING HOUSE CALLS.

SAMPLE NEWS RELEASE

Following is an example of a news release created at a media relations seminar with family physicians/researchers at the Thames Valley Family Practice Research Unit in London, Ontario. We attempted to follow as many of the points as possible mentioned above in "The Characteristics of a Good News Release."

```
             FAMILY MEDICINE NEWSLINK
             "FOR IMMEDIATE RELEASE"

                                    London, Ontario
                                    November 19, 1992

       PATIENTS WANT TO KNOW MORE ABOUT WHAT AILS THEM

         Patients expect family doctors to give them good
    information  concerning  health  problems  and  how  to
```

manage them. A recent study involving 20 family physicians (a mix of urban and rural) and 400 patients found that the most common topics patients want to know about are high blood pressure, neck pain, cholesterol levels, headache, sore throats, and diabetes.

On the whole, family physicians do a good job communicating information to patients, according to the study. More than 90% of the patients say they are very satisfied with information given, and 85% understand it well. But almost one in four patients say they still have further questions about their condition after their appointment.

"Although it's gratifying to learn that patients and doctors appear to communicate well with each other, the study shows there is still lots of room for improvement," says Dr. I. Care of the Family Practice Research Unit in Healthy, Ontario. "We need to sense when there might be questions we haven't covered."

When asked whether they prefer verbal explanations, printed handouts, diagrams or models, audio or video tapes, or information concerning groups or programs, most patients want additional verbal explanations or printed pamphlets.

"Even when patients felt their needs for information had been dealt with satisfactorily, more than a third said they also would have liked a book about their condition and many also said they wanted a videotape," Dr. Care says. "As physicians we need to be willing to try a variety of communications approaches."

Maintaining clear, supportive doctor-patient communication is as important as making a correct diagnosis, Dr. Care observes. Good communications are crucial to the model of shared decision making that increasingly plays an central role in today's medical practices.

For more information on doctors communicating health care information to patients, contact Dr. I. Care at the Family Practice Research Unit, (000) 123-4567.

ANALYSIS OF THE SAMPLE NEWS RELEASE

1. *FAMILY MEDICINE NEWSLINK*—This is an example of a heading that could be included on news releases printed on stationery from the Thames Valley Family Practice Research Unit. The words "FOR IMMEDIATE RELEASE" go directly under, followed by city and date.

2. *PATIENTS WANT TO KNOW MORE ABOUT WHAT AILS THEM*— Headline indicates what the news release is about and arouses reader's interest (e.g., What is the "more"? Are we not being told enough?).

3. *Paragraph 1*—Gives the bottom-line information of the study—that patients expect good information and more of it. This is the "lead," and is followed by a brief description of the research study.

4. *Paragraph 2*—Gives a general impression of the study and makes use of three key statistics—the 90% of patients who said they were satisfied, the 85% who said they understood the information well, and the one in four who still have questions.

5. *Paragraph 3*—A quote from a key source for the research study. This identifies who the source is. The more conversational tone introduced at this point moves the story forward.

6. *Paragraph 4*—Provides a little more information on patients' expectations and needs concerning communications, but the paragraph is kept very brief.

7. *Paragraph 5*—A second quote from the source conveys further significant information and arrives at a conclusion. Putting this information in quote form helps give the news release more "voice" than if it were simply presented as an informational paragraph.

8. *Paragraph 6*—Alludes to the wider significance of the research study, why it was done, and what the direction of the future is likely to be.

9. *Paragraph 7*—Names the person quoted in the article as the contact person for the press. This indicates that this person is willing to be interviewed and has the additional information required to flesh out the news story.

If You Are Contacted by the Media

If as a result of issuing a news release, you are contacted by a reporter for an interview, the news release is an excellent basis upon which to start, because the reporter already has your reader-friendly, accurate information in hand.

It does also happen, however, that medical researchers and physicians are called out of the blue by members of the press seeking a comment on a current news issue or controversy. Or it may be someone who is doing a story—for example, on head-aches—and wants to tap your knowledge of the subject. There are some strategies you can follow to avoid being caught totally off guard and to increase the odds of a useful interview that will not be misquoted.

1. Find out the reporter's name, the publication/broadcast station for which he or she works, and who the target audience is.

2. Be accessible. If the interview is going to be fairly substantial, do it face to face, not on the telephone (for shorter interviews, a telephone conversation is fine). Recognize the deadline pressure on the re-porter in agreeing on a time for the interview.

3. If you have set a time for an interview, write down in advance the points you would like to make. If you are called on the spot and do not feel comfortable thinking on your feet, ask the reporter to call back (or be called back) in about 10 minutes, and use this time to jot down some points. If you have been caught at an inconvenient time, decide on a mutually agreeable time to talk.

4. As with the printed news release, keep the verbal interview conver-sational and avoid professional jargon. Do not bombard the reporter with statistics, but do help him or her to understand the situation better by providing useful background information.

5. If you are asked to comment on an unfamiliar area, it is acceptable to say something like "This is not an issue I'm familiar with," or "I would need to know more about the subject before I could venture an opinion."

6. Do not speak "off the record"—assume that every statement you make could become part of the story. Also, do not say "no comment" because this suggests you are hiding something.

7. If the story is for the public media, you will not have the right to see it before it is printed or broadcast. You can, however, ask if the information is to be fact-checked and who will be doing the checking.

If You Are "On the Air"

ON THE AIR ON RADIO

A very popular way of interviewing medical professionals is by radio. Radio is the most interactive of all the media, in that through live interviews and "phone-in" public input, it has a sense of immediacy that other media lack.

Some tips for being interviewed on the radio:

1. If you know ahead of time that you are to be interviewed live on radio, it is appropriate to discuss with the show's host or interviewer what questions you will be asked to respond to. The big fear in "going live" is not knowing what to say on the spot. Knowing in advance what is going to be covered in the interview, although not a guarantee that you will perform confidently, at least takes the edge off preinterview jitters.

2. Remember, one of radio's main mandates is to *entertain* listeners. Be prepared for the interviewer's attempt to inject some humor or wit into the interview (unless it is a subject where it would be in bad taste to do so). Often, a radio interviewer will ask about something the two of you have not previously discussed (the "out-of-left-field" question); if you agree to be interviewed on radio, you must be prepared to field spontaneous questions.

ON THE AIR ON TV

1. TV interviewers usually give some indication ahead of time of what the questions will be. The issue to be aware of with television is that you may do an hour-long interview, and then only a few minutes (sometimes even less than a minute) of the interview will be included in the final broadcast. Even if it is an extended documentary interview, there will be parts that will not get into the broadcast. You have no control over the editing process or the decision as to which "sound bite" will be used. As with print, when the cameras roll, assume that everything you say could potentially end up on the screen, so do not speak off the record.

2. TV station staff are usually happy to give you advice on how to dress for an on-camera interview. Wear your most flattering colors, but definitely avoid bright "busy" patterns, such as a vibrant colored plaid. Solid colors work best on TV; if you wear more than one color, ask someone who knows you if your look "goes together" visually.

Responding to What Patients
Have Read or Seen in the Media

One aspect of media relations that is seldom considered, but very widespread, is what to do when patients bring information they have seen in media stories to their physicians. For example, a patient wants a prescription for a new drug, or has read conflicting reports (e.g., one article suggesting that totally abstaining from alcohol is most healthy, and another suggesting that moderate drinking may have beneficial health effects such as improving circulation).

If you have not seen the article in question, you will have no sense of the story's factuality or its context. Yet because, as Peter Desbarats points out in Chapter 6, patients glean much of their health information from media coverage, simply dismissing the patient's interest does not create a good climate for doctor-patient communication. As yet there is little research on the effect of media information on this communication, but here are some approaches physicians might take:

1. Ideally, if the patient has brought the article in, take some time to look at it together. If what is claimed in the article sounds too good to be true, stress to the patient that it probably is too good to be true.

2. Often the patient will not have the article. If you have not seen it, say so, and state that you cannot comment appropriately on something you have not read but that you are willing to look at it. Ask the patient to bring it in or send it to you.

3. If it is a question of a new drug or treatment, offer to find out accurate information from a reliable source; then you can discuss with the patient whether or not it is potentially useful for his or her specific condition.

4. Help patients identify where they themselves can get further information. For example, if the patient has seen a TV broadcast about young children being immunized against meningitis and wants to know more, there may be a pamphlet you can provide. You could also direct patients to a source such as the public health unit. If the article or TV show was about heart disease, you could encourage them to get more information from the Heart and Stroke Foundation in Canada or the American Heart Association.

5. Keep a good supply in your office of up-to-date pamphlets and articles that contain what you consider to be reliable information.

6. Perhaps medical professionals—locally, state-wide or provincially, or even nationally—could begin a "media watch," creating short summaries of what major publications and TV shows are covering on medicine.

Index

Abstracts, 54-55, 56, 166
  structured, 56, 88
Academic detailing, 11-12, 145, 146,
  148, 181, 182
Adult learning theory, 6, 7, 99
Advertising, 4, 7
Agency for Health Care Policy and Re-
  search (AHCPR), 98, 155, 190, 208
Ambulatory Sentinel Practice Network
  (ASPN), 47, 159,
Audit, 47, 101, 164, 168, 170, 174, 175
  chart, 4, 129, 147, 148, 168
  feedback from, 13
Authorship, 38, 56, 72-73, 91, 131, 133

Behavior change, 8, 11, 13, 41, 100, 146,
  155, 165
  affecting patient care, 41
  of physicians, 5-10, 15, 33, 41, 50,
  106, 139-210
Biomedical research, 46, 156, 157, 158,
  214

Canadian National Research System
  (NARES), 159
Change, 25, 97, 98, 110, 112, 120, 147,
  148, 188
  acceptance of, 8, 106
  agents, 98, 145
  economic incentives for, 13
  methods for evaluating, 115-121

motivators for, 5, 6, 147
  process of, 106, 110, 120, 175
Chart review. *See* Audit
Clinical decision making, 2, 3, 5, 11, 14,
  163, 164, 170
Clinical policies, 151-161, 167, 170, 187,
  203. *See also* Guidelines, Policies
  and physician behavior, 151, 152,
  155-158, 170, 187
  and research, 159-160
Clinical practice, influences on, 152-
  154, 155-158, 160, 162, 180, 199
Collaboration, 10, 104
Communication, 21-30, 76, 77, 78, 93
  among researchers, 22-23
  attributes of, 7
  between researchers and policy
  makers, 25-27, 208-209
  between researchers and practitioners, 23-25
  between researchers, media and the
  public, 27-28, 78, 206, 213
  definition of, 21
  networks, 21, 29, 98
  of research findings, 7, 13, 51
  persuasive, 7, 8
  physician-patient, 13, 217, 221
  problems of, 26, 77, 78
Community, 10, 14, 127, 128, 131, 132,
  133
  forums, 133, 134
Computers, 12, 142, 146, 164, 166, 168,
  195

223

About the Editors

Earl V. Dunn (MD) is Professor in both the Department of Family and Community Medicine and the Centre for Studies in Medical Education at the University of Toronto. His research centers on medical decision making, telemedicine, resource utilization, and the economics of health care delivery. He has published in all these fields.

Peter G. Norton (PhD, MD) is Associate Professor in the Department of Family and Community Medicine at the University of Toronto and Vice President of Medicine, Psychiatry, and Long Term Care at Sunnybrook Health Science Centre in Toronto. His research specialties include medical decision making, utilization of health care resources, alternative models of health care delivery, and research methodologies for primary care.

Moira Stewart (PhD) is Professor in the Department of Family Medicine and the Centre for Studies in Family Medicine at The University of Western Ontario, London, Ontario, Canada. She is an Epidemiologist who for the past 15 years has applied her research skills to two general topics: stress in relation to health and communication between patients and doctors. She has published numerous articles in *Social Science and Medicine, Medical Care, Family Practice: An International Journal, Canadian Medical Association Journal, Journal of the Royal College of General Practitioners,* and the *British Medical Journal.* She has been particularly active in fostering an international network of teachers and scientists of communication in medicine through the International Conference on Doctor–Patient Communication, the American Academy, and the North American Primary Care Research Group's Interest Group on Doctor–Patient Communication. She has edited two books, *Communicating With Medical Patients* and *Tools for Primary Care Research* and is coauthor of *Patient-Centered Communication: Theory, Research and Education* (forthcoming).

Fred Tudiver (MD) is Associate Professor in the Department of Family and Community Medicine at Sunnybrook Health Science Centre and the University of Toronto. His research interests include health promotion including the application of self-help and mutual group support techniques, men's health issues, and primary care counseling and psychology.

Martin J. Bass (MD) is Director of the Centre for Studies in Family Medicine at The University of Western Ontario. He was the sole Canadian and the only family physician to be appointed as one of 29 Kellogg International Fellows. His research interests include hypertension in family practice, natural history of headaches, technology application in family practice, prevention, and quality of care. He is past Chairman of the National Research Committee of the College of Family Physicians of Canada and is the current holder of the McWhinney Chair for Research in Family Medicine.

About the Contributors

John Bain (MD) was formerly a general practitioner in Livingston New Town in Scotland and a Senior Lecturer in General Practice in the University of Aberdeen. He was Head of the Department of Primary Medical Care at Aldermoor Health Centre, Southampton, for 10 years before taking up his present post as Professor of General Practice at Tayside Centre for General Practice in Dundee. His research interests have focused on two broad areas: respiratory illness in children, and management development in general practice. He is actively involved in educational programs for medical students and trainee practitioners and is one of those responsible for creating an integrated department of undergraduate and postgraduate general practice. He has recently studied and reported on the effect of health care reforms on the delivery of primary medical care in the United Kingdom.

Renaldo N. Battista (MD, ScD) is Director of the Division of Clinical Epidemiology, Montreal General Hospital, and Associate Professor in Epidemiology and Biostatistics, Family Medicine, and Medicine at McGill University. He has an MD from the University of Montreal, and an MPH and ScD in Health Policy and Management, both from Harvard University. He is Vice-Chairman of the Canadian Task Force on the Periodic Health Examination, a member of Quebec's Council on Health Care Technology Assessment, and a member of the Board of the International Society of Technology Assessment in Health Care.

Richard Birtwhistle (MD) is Associate Professor of Family Medicine and Assistant Professor of Community Health and Epidemiology at Queen's University, Kingston, Ontario. He is also Director of Clinical Skills Program in the Faculty of Medicine. His current research interests are in teaching communication and clinical skills to medical students, the use of screening tests in family practice, and follow-up visits in chronic disease.

Marilyn Bookbinder (RN, PhD) is Acting Director of Nursing Research at Memorial Sloan-Kettering Cancer Center. She is Adjunct Associate Professor at New York University and Columbia University and is a member of the Board of Trustees for the New York City Metropolitan Library Association. She is on the editorial board of *Oncology Nursing Forum* and *Applied Nursing Research.* Her research interests include research utilization and evaluating the impact of implementing national pain management guidelines in a comprehensive cancer center. She is currently collaborating with New York University studying the adjustment of couples following breast cancer and with Columbia University examining nurses' job stress and menstrual functioning. Her publications reflect these areas of interest.

David A. Davis (MD) is a fellow of the College of Family Physicians of Canada and is Associate Dean of Continuing Medical Education at the University of Toronto. In addition, he is a Professor in the Department of Family and Community Medicine of the University of Toronto. He is interested in the patterns of physician learning, the determinants of physician competence, and the effectiveness of continuing medical education (CME), and has researched, published, and spoken widely in these related areas. He is a member of and has served in leadership positions in several provincial, national, and North American organizations related to CME, including the Ontario Council for CME, the Standing Committee for CME of the Association of Canadian Medical Colleges, the Society of Medical College Directors of CME, and the Alliance for CME.

Peter Desbarats has been Dean of the Graduate School of Journalism at The University of Western Ontario since 1981. During three decades in journalism, he worked for print and broadcast media in Canada and overseas. His nine published books include political and historical works as well as children's books. His most recent work is *Guide to Canadian News Media* (1990). In 1980-1981, he was Senior Consultant and Associate Research Director with the Royal Commission on Newspapers where he authored a published study on the impact of new information technologies on Canadian newspapers. He is the founding president of an association of directors of journalism programs at Canadian Universities. In 1986, he directed a study of news programming for the Federal Task Force on Broadcasting Policy. He researched political communication for the 1992 Royal Commission on Electoral Reform. In 1992 he was a member of the Ontario government's Task Force on Cardiovascular Services. He is a member of the Communications Advisory Committee for UNESCO in Canada, the Editorial Board of the *Canadian Journal of Communications,* the Selection Committee for the Canadian News Hall of Fame, and regularly acts as a judge in national competitions for magazine and newspaper journalism, radio and television journalism, and investigative journalism.

Allen J. Dietrich (MD), Professor of Community and Family Medicine, is the senior academic family physician at Dartmouth Medical School, an active primary care researcher, and a member of the Dartmouth Primary Care Cooperative Information Project (COOP). Through the Cancer Prevention in Community Practice Project, he has worked with community practices in New Hampshire, Vermont, and federally sponsored Community Health Centers for the underserved in New York and New Jersey to assist them in enhancing the cancer early detection and prevention services they provide. These projects provide a database on 15,000 patients, more than 60 community health centers, and more than 200 community practices. His major research interests include the process by which innovations are adopted into primary care practices and nontraditional evaluation methods such as standardized patients. In addition to his research, he is Director of Undergraduate Family Medicine Education and Director of Clinical Symposia, a first-year required course that provides a clinical foundation for the basic science learning of medical students. He has maintained a community practice for 11 years in Lebanon, NH.

Tom Elmslie (MD, MSc, CCFP, FRCPC) is Associate Professor of Family Medicine and of Community Medicine and Epidemiology at the University of Ottawa, Vice-Chair for Research of the Department of Family Medicine; and Director of the Clinical Epidemiology Unit, Elisabeth Bruyere Health Centre. He is active in the College of Family Physicians of Canada where he is a member of the National Research Committee; Chair of the planning committee of the National Research Systems (NaReS); and a member of the steering committee for the Clinical Guidelines Project. He received his medical undergraduate training at McMaster University and completed his residency in family medicine at the University of Ottawa. Over the past 4 years he has Chaired the Ottawa Family Medicine Department's working group on evidence-based family medicine, developing and implementing this curriculum in the residency program. He has recently become involved in establishing an evidence-based medicine component in the first 2 years of the undergraduate medical program.

Azana N. Endicott (BA) is a Research Coordinator at the Department of Clinical Epidemiology at the Montreal General Hospital and at the Royal Victoria Hospital in Montreal, Canada. She also produces two radio current affairs shows. She studied English literature and journalism at Queen's University in Kingston and Concordia University in Montreal. Her main research interests is the coverage of health care issues in the media.

Vivek Goel (MD, CM, MSc, SM) is a Scientist with the Institute for Clinical Evaluative Sciences in Ontario and the Clinical Epidemiology Unit, Sunnybrook Health Science Centre, as well as an Assistant Professor in the Department of Preventive Medicine and

Biostatistics. He is also an Associate Member of the Graduate Department of Community Health at the University of Toronto. He obtained his MD from McGill University, completed an internship at St. Joseph's Health Centre in Toronto, worked for one year as a general practitioner in Ontario, and then entered the Community Medicine Residency Program at the University of Toronto. He completed an MS in Health Administration with a focus in Health Policy and Health Economics at the University of Toronto, followed by an MSc in Biostatistics with a focus in Health Decision Sciences at the Harvard School of Public Health. He is a Fellow of the Royal College of Physicians of Canada in Community Medicine. His current research interests focus on the evaluation of health services, particularly the accessibility of services. He has a special interest in the examination of preventive health services.

Larry A. Green (MD) is Professor and Woodward-Chisholm Chairman of the Department of Family Practice at the University of Colorado. He is a graduate of Baylor College of Medicine and completed his residency training in Family Practice at the University of Rochester and Highland Hospital in 1976. He is a member of the founding Board of Directors of the Ambulatory Sentinel Practice Network (ASPN) and has been active in the work of ASPN as well as the development of other practice-based research networks, both in North America and abroad. He participated in the development of the International Primary Care Network (IPCN) and serves on its Board of Directors. As an active participant in national efforts to promote family practice in the United States, he has served on the Board of Directors of the Association of Departments of Family Medicine and of the North American Primary Care Research Group. He is a member of the editorial board of the *Journal of the American Board of Family Practice* and has been an active contributor to the literature with numerous articles relating to practice-based research. In 1991 he was elected to membership in the Institute of Medicine of the National Academy of Sciences. He is a member of the American Academy of Family Practice and is a Diplomate of the American Board of Family Practice.

Carol P. Herbert (MD) is Royal Canadian Legion Professor and Head of the Department of Family Practice at the University of British Columbia. She is certificant and Fellow of the College of Family Physicians of Canada. She has been the YWCA Woman of Distinction in Health and Social Sciences, a member of the National Research Committee, Chair of the B.C. Chapter Research Committee, and Chair of the NRC and President of the Board of NAPCRG. Her research questions have been spawned by her practice experience. Her current research is focused on assault and sexual abuse, and the development of community-based research.

Penny Jennett (PhD) trained in Regina Grey Nun's Hospital in Regina, Saskatchewan, before practicing as a professional health record administrator for several years in acute care hospitals in Saskatoon, and psychiatric facilities across Canada. She worked with the College of Physicians and Surgeons of Saskatchewan and the College of Medicine at the University of Saskatchewan as a research assistant and research associate over a 10-year period on various activities studying how physicians and future physicians practice and learn. She earned her master's and PhD in Medical Education at the College of Human Medicine at Michigan State University. After the completion of her doctorate she returned to the province of Saskatchewan to work on a 3-year continuing medical education research project funded by Health and Welfare Canada. At this time she was selected to be the first PhD within a faculty of medicine to be awarded a $75,000 scholarship by the Canadian Life and Health Association. She is currently Associate Professor and Director of the Office of Medical Education at the Faculty of Medicine in Calgary. Her wide range of research interests include practice culture, medical informatics, health economics, and medical manpower issues.

Roger Jones (MA, DM, BM, Beh) is Wolfson Professor of General Practice at UMDS (Guy's and St. Thomas' Hospitals). He has held previous posts in academic primary care in Southampton and Newcastle upon Tyne. His main area of research interest over the past 10 years has been in the epidemiology, natural history, and management of common gastrointestinal problems; this research has acted as the basis for a number of other interests, principally in the interface between primary and secondary care, in clinical decision making and in the dissemination and implementation of research findings to service practice. He edits *Family Practice*, an international journal of primary health care published by Oxford University Press, and is an active member of the British Society of Gastroenterology and Chairman of the Primary Care Society for Gastroenterology. As Secretary of the Heads of Departments group of the Association of University Departments of General Practice in the United Kingdom, he is involved in curriculum review and innovation and in the development of primary care as an academic discipline.

Jacques Lemelin (MD) is Assistant Professor and clinical researcher in the Clinical Epidemiology Unit of the Department of Family Medicine, University of Ottawa, and Research Coordinator at the Melrose Family Medicine Unit. He is presently in the process of setting up a primary care community-based research network in Ottawa. Prior to joining the Department of Family Medicine, he practiced rural family medicine for 13 years. His research interests include depression and medical informatics.

Sharon Lindenburger is a journalist, author, scriptwriter, editor, and researcher specializing in health care, biomedical research, science and technology, the environment, and education. She is coauthor (with Philip Hassen, CEO of St. Joseph's Health Centre, London) of the book *Rx for Hospitals: New Hope for Medicare in the Nineties* (1993). She has written feature articles in a wide variety of publications—both for the health care sector and in the public media—on topics such as pregnancy and birth, issues of aging, future trends in health care, community approaches to health, and quality in health care. She is a former secondary school teacher and adult educator, has conducted media literacy workshops for elementary and secondary school students, and has taught adult credit courses in English, including media awareness. She also works with many health care professionals on developing communication strategies for the dissemination of research findings and other important health care information to the general public.

Jonathan Lomas (BA, MA) grew up in Great Britain and did his undergraduate training in experimental psychology at Oxford University. He came to Canada in 1973 as a Commonwealth Scholar doing further study in psychology at The University of Western Ontario. His background since that time includes work or training in health economics, political science, and epidemiology with the University of Toronto and the Canadian Political Science Association. He is currently a Professor of Health Policy Analysis in the Department of Clinical Epidemiology and Biostatistics, and the Coordinator of the Centre for Health Economics and Policy Analysis at McMaster University. He is also one of the Ontario Ministry of Health's Career Scientists and an Associate of the Population Health Programme of the Canadian Institute for Advanced Research. He has published two books and numerous articles and chapters in the areas of health policy and health services research. His main interest is in the impact and transfer of evidence for decision making. He has done research on methods for manpower planning, alternative funding and organizational arrangements for the delivery of care, quality assurance, practice guidelines and their implementation, and the determinants of clinical policies in areas such as obstetrical care and cardiovascular disease. His main interest currently is in evaluating local health and social service decision making.

Eric M. Meslin (PhD) is the Assistant Director, University of Toronto Centre for Bioethics and Associate Director of the Clinical Ethics Centre at Sunnybrook Health Science Centre. He is also Assistant Professor of Philosophy at the University of Toronto, and is cross-appointed in the Faculty of Medicine, the Faculty of Pharmacy, and the Department of Health Administration. He holds an undergraduate degree in Philosophy from York University and received his MA and PhD from the Bioethics Program in Philosophy at the Kennedy Institute of Ethics at Georgetown University in Washington, DC. Before coming to Sunnybrook in

1988, he was a Program Analyst in the Office for Protection from Research Risks at the National Institutes of Health in Bethesda, Maryland, and from 1985-1987 he directed the Research Ethics Program at the American Psychological Association in Washington, DC. At Sunnybrook, he serves as the hospital's bioethicist, providing clinical and research consultation, conducting research in bioethics, and teaching staff and students. At the Centre for Bioethics, his research interests include: advance directives, the ethics of resource allocation in the Canadian health care system, and medical research ethics. He lectures widely on ethical issues in medicine, research, and health policy and has published on topics such as medical research ethics, death and dying, and physician reimbursement. He is the current Chair of Sunnybrook's Research Board, a member of several Hospital Ethics Committees, and a member of the Board of Directors of the Multiple Organ Retrieval and Exchange Program of Ontario.

Janice M. Morse (PhD) is Professor of Nursing and Behavioral Science at the School of Nursing, College of Health and Human Development, The Pennsylvania State University. With doctorates in both nursing and anthropology, she conducts research into patient care, in particular into patient comfort, patient falls, and patient restraints; into women's health issues, such as menarche, childbirth, and breast-feeding; and cross-cultural health. She has published more than 100 articles, authored and coauthored several books, including *Qualitative Nursing Research: A Contemporary Dialogue* and, with Joy Johnson, *The Illness Experience: Dimensions of Suffering,* and is the editor of an international multidisciplinary journal, *Qualitative Health Research.*

C. David Naylor (MD, DPhil) is Chief Executive Officer, Institute for Clinical Evaluative Sciences in Ontario, and Director of the Clinical Epidemiology Program, Sunnybrook Health Science Centre. Educated at the University of Toronto, he graduated with scholarships in medicine, surgery, and paediatrics in 1978. He traveled to Oxford as a Rhodes Scholar, receiving a DPhil in social and administrative sciences in 1983. He is on staff in general internal medicine at Sunnybrook and an Associate Professor in the Department of Medicine at the University of Toronto. He is Principal Investigator on the ICES Project, a 5-year special award from the Ministry of Health that has provided $20.5 million in operating funds, as well as a major capital award, for development of a health services research facility. He participates in various projects funded by the Institute, including a trial to improve drug utilization in the management of acute myocardial infarction, a before-after comparison of patterns of X-ray use after implementation of an algorithm for clinical examination of patients with suspected ankle fractures, and a study to examine the implementation of advance directives for dialysis patients. As a second-term career scientist of the Ontario Ministry of Health, his independent research has been in the realm of cardiovascular disease, particularly at the interface of clinical epidemiology and public policy. He has authored or coauthored more than 100 scholarly articles, book chapters, technical reports, and monographs.

Kathleen F. Norr (PhD) is a Medical Sociologist at the College of Nursing, University of Illinois at Chicago. She has a strong interest in the primary health-care model as a way to improve health care for women and children in both developed and developing countries. She is currently conducting an evaluation of a primary health-care based program for low-income mothers in Chicago. She is also committed to the use of the primary health-care model for AIDS prevention for women internationally. She is currently evaluating a peer education intervention for AIDS prevention among women in Botswana. She is also interested in the process of birth and ways in which the birth process can be made safe and satisfying for women and their families. She is currently conducting observation of labor support in a tertiary care setting by different types of care providers with Dr. Joyce Roberts.

Paul A. Nutting (MD, MSPH) is Professor of Family Medicine at the University of Colorado Health Sciences Center and Director of the Ambulatory Sentinel Practice Network. He was educated at Cornell University, received his MD degree from the University of

Kansas, and an MS in Epidemiology and Biometry from the University of Colorado. He has residency training in Family Medicine at the Mercy Medical Center in Denver, Pediatrics at the Children's Hospital of Pittsburgh, and Preventive Medicine at the University of Arizona. He is certified by the American Board of Family Practice and by the American Board of Preventive Medicine. He formerly served with the U.S. Public Health Service as Deputy Director of the Center for General Health Services Research and the Director of the Division of Primary Care for the Agency for Health Care Policy and Research. Prior to that he served as Director of Research for the Indian Health Service and as the Director of the Office of Primary Care Studies in the Health Resources and Services Administration. He also spent 2 years as a Senior Scholar-in-Residence at the Institute of Medicine of the National Academy of Science. He is on the editorial board of *The American Family Physician* and *The Journal of Family Practice,* and has previously served on the board of the *Journal of Community Health.*

Emily A. C. Ruiz (MD, PhD), earned her MSc from the University of London and her PhD from the Public Health School of Sao Paulo University, Brazil. Her experience in the field of health care has mainly been as a health care administrator and as a researcher in the health care field at the Sao Paulo State Health Secretariat. Her main research interests are in quality assurance and human resources in health care services.

Yves Talbot (MD) is Associate Professor in Family Medicine, Pediatrics and Health Administration. He practices Family Medicine and is the Coordinator of the Research Programs in Family Medicine at the University of Toronto. He was a Robert Wood Johnson Scholar at McGill University and the University of Pennsylvania. He was a faculty member at the Kellogg Centre for Advanced Studies in Primary Care (McGill). His research and scholarly interests have been mainly in family and education.

Kerr Lachlan White (MD) was Deputy Director for Health Sciences of the Rockefeller Foundation from 1978-1984. From 1964 to

1977 he was Professor of Health Care Organization and founding chairman of that department at the Johns Hopkins University. He was educated at McGill University in economics, political science, and medicine, and did postgraduate work at Yale University, the London Hospital Medical School, and the London School of Hygiene and Tropical Medicine. In addition to a residency in internal medicine, a fellowship year at McGill included training in psychiatry. For a decade he practiced and taught internal medicine at the University of North Carolina with a special emphasis on psychosocial aspects of care, including research on the influence of emotional factors on venous pressure and congestive heart failure. During that period he introduced the term *primary medical care* and conducted a number of early studies in the field that was later defined as "Health Service Research." He is the author or coauthor of more than 200 publications, including 10 books, in the fields of health services, health statistics, epidemiology, public health, and medical education, including *Epidemiology as a Fundamental Science; Health Care: An International Study; The Task of Medicine,* and *Health the Schism.*

Marjorie L. Wood (MD) is Assistant Professor in Family Medicine at The University of Western Ontario. She was born in Scotland and graduated in medicine from the University of Glasgow in 1967. Following postgraduate training in pediatrics, obstetrics and gynecology in Edinburgh she emigrated to Canada in 1970. After initial work in family practice she was Employee Health Physician at University Hospital, London, from 1973 to 1983 where she was instrumental in setting up employee assistance and rehabilitation programs. From 1983 to 1988 she was Clinical Associate at the London Regional Cancer Centre working with breast cancer patients and setting up a community-based Palliative Care Team. In 1988, she renewed her interest in family medicine, spending 6 months in the postgraduate program then going on to graduate from the Masters in Clinical Science program, both at The University of Western Ontario. In the latter program she pursued an interest in cancer patient care in family practice and has done research work in the area of communication between oncologists and family physicians in cancer patient care. From 1990 to 1993 she was Liaison Physician to the Thames Valley Family Practice Research Unit and continues as a member of the family physician partners of the Unit. Since 1990, she has been in private family practice with particular interests in palliative care, cancer patient care, and home-based care. Additional interests include encouraging family physicians to become involved in practice-based research and writing for medical journals.